*Mr Settles, Thank you have control of everyone associated with The UAW
God bless you
Dolores Jackson*

Healing the Hurts of Yesterday

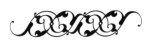

Dolores Jackson

Healing the Hurts of Yesterday

By Dolores Jackson
© 2016 Dolores Jackson
Printed in the United States of America
ISBN 978-1533429766

All rights reserved sole by the author. The author guarantees all contents are original and do not infringe upon the legal rights of any other person or work. No part of this book may be reproduced, stored in a retrieval system, or transmitted in any form or by any means without expressed written permission of the author.

Habakkuk Publishing
Canton, Michigan

Editor:

Printed in the U.S.A.

DEDICATION

This book is dedicated to my heavenly Father. All honor, glory and praise belong to you Lord God. Thank you so much for giving me this great gift to be able to communicate what is in your heart, and on your mind through writing, and for giving me the strength to endure and continue on even when I didn't think I had it in me to go further. Thank you for speaking through me, for all that you have imparted in me, and for the opportunity to do something that is truly for the good of all people. It is an honor to know you, to serve you, and to be chosen by you to do such a great work.

    I would like to thank my mother for being such a great inspiration to me, for your love and support, and for being the best mother that anyone could ever have. I love you so much.

    Thanks to my sister Yvonne, my granddaughter Iyana, and to my best friends Kyra and Sanja, for all of the support, and encouragement, and for helping to pray me through the process of writing this book.

    I would like to thank my father in the spirit Bishop Willie M. Thornton for taking the time to impart knowledge, wisdom, understanding, and the principles of God's word into my life. I have learned so much under your tutor ledge, and I look forward to everything that I have yet to learn from you.

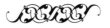

TABLE OF CONTENTS

Dedication iii

Introduction 1

Chapter 1: The Origin of Pain 3

Chapter 2: Understanding the Complexity of the Heart 9

Chapter 3: You Are Not Alone 15

Chapter 4: Unmasking the Pain 21

Chapter 5: Pushing Past the Pain 27

Chapter 6: Identifying the Source of Your Pain 33

      Medical Clause 38

Chapter 7: Understanding the Source 39

Chapter 8: Addictions 43

      Cutting & Self-harm 43

      Gambling addiction/problem gambling 53

      Pornography Addiction 70

      Sexual Addiction 75

Chapter 9: Substance Abuse Addiction 81

      Alcohol Abuse/Alcoholism 81

      Smoking Cessation 84

      Street and Prescription Drugs 90

Chapter 10: Mental Health Illnesses 99

    Anxiety 99

    Bipolar Disorder 106

    Depression 113

    Eating Disorders Anorexia Nervosa 121

    Binge Eating 132

    Bulimia Nervosa 142

    Obsessive Compulsive Disorder (OCD) 151

    Post-Traumatic Stress Disorder (PTSD) 161

    Schizoid Personality Disorder 170

    Schizophrenia 173

Chapter 11: Emotional and Psychological Trauma 185

    Abandonment 187

    Caregiver Burnout Stress 192

    Child Abuse and Neglect 199

    Divorce/ Breakup 214

    Domestic Violence and Abuse 225

    Elderly Abuse 236

    Stress 244

Glossary 255

About the Author 283

INTRODUCTION

FROM THE TIME we enter into this world we are taught the basics of life, and as children we are very vulnerable and so full of life and joy. As we grow up our earliest memories are those of what we experience in our homes, and they have the greatest influence on us. They ultimately set the stage for the type of person we will be, what we will believe, how we will treat others, what our view point in life will be and what kind of relationships we will enter into. As children we are sheltered having no real understanding of what lies beyond the front door of our home or what lies ahead of us as we set off to embark upon the life we were created to live. As we go out into the world we know nothing except what we are taught by our parents, and if we are not properly prepared before leaving home it will have us at a great disadvantage.

Unfortunately, no matter how much training we receive from our parents, all of us are subject to vulnerabilities and this is something that we can't escape. We were taught to walk in love, to try and get along with others, and that if we are good to others, they will in turn be good to us. So we take this mindset into the world with us believing this is true, only to find that it is the furthest thing from the truth. This is not because our parents taught us in error, but it is because a great portion of the world does not live by the same principles. So as we embark upon our journey in life, we quickly find that there are many things in this world that we are not prepared for, and that life, no matter how painful it may be, is just a training ground where we are learning how to be responsible and productive individuals.

In this life we will find that two of the strongest feelings we will ever encounter is love and pain, and that it will be determined which of the two will out way the other in our lives, through our own strengths and weaknesses, how well we can stand up under pressure, and also which of the two we've been exposed to the most. It is unfortunate but as children we are prepared to receive and experience love, but not pain. We are taught to live in peace, but we are not taught that in life we will have to fight many wars, nor are we prepared for the time they would come. And we are taught not to hurt others, but we are not taught that even though it may not always be intentional, at some point they will surely hurt us. There are billions of hurting people in this world, that need to know that they are not alone in what they're going through, and that their pain can in many cases be a help to them rather than a hindrance, or a death sentence. I would like to take you on a journey me, that I believe will help you understand where your pain originated from, help you understand how to deal with it, and ultimately learn how to get past it and move on with your life. But in the meantime it is more important at the beginning of all this for you to know, that though it may feel like your pain is going to kill you it won't, and also though it won't happen overnight, it is possible for you to overcome your pain, and brokenness and be healed from all of your past hurts.

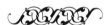

CHAPTER 1

The Origin of Pain

PAIN IS SOMETHING that everyone on earth has experienced to some degree or another, whether it was from a love relationship, a friendship, family relationship, loss of a job, sickness and disease, etc.

The first thing you need to understand is that there are different types of pain, and there are different levels of pain. The definition for pain is bodily or mental suffering. Both can be temporary or permanent, both can be masked with medicine and both can be devastating, having a lasting affect on your life and can range from a minor pain, having minimal affects, to pain that is very deeply felt and can have a major impact on your life.

Bodily suffering can be caused by injury, or surgery, and while it can be very serious and difficult to deal with, it can be masked with pain medicine and over a period of time can either heal or be managed. But then you have pain that is caused by illnesses that can be chronic, or acute. Chronic pain is generally associated with long-term illness, and this kind of pain can be very persistent and may linger for many years. Acute pain is usually associated with illnesses that are severe and lasts only a short duration of time, and this kind of pain though short lived can be just as devastating depending upon the severity of it. When dealing with extreme pain for both short and long periods of time, it can begin to affect you mentally, and can be even more devastating, because when dealing with situations such as this at some point it will also begin to affect you emotionally.

The second type of pain is mental suffering, and depending upon how long this mental distress lasts and the level of it, it can eventually lead to emotional illnesses, such as Depression, Bi-polar, and even schizophrenia. Mental suffering can have an even greater effect on you, because the pain is trapped on the inside of you rather than just being a surface pain, it is not as easy to escape, requires a different type of medicine as well as the need for counseling, and sometimes hospitalization and this medicine as well as other medicine can cause an entirely separate issue. Though these types of diseases may not cause physical pain, they are still very painful and have the ability to not only destroy your life, but also to cause you to become a prisoner of your own mind. These diseases can ruin relationships, cause you to have difficulty in concentrating and solving simple everyday problems, and can also cause you to have feelings of guilt and worthlessness, and even thoughts of suicide. Emotional suffering can be brought on by things such as worrying, bad relationships, mental and physical abuse, incarceration, rape, stress, loss of a loved one, and etc.

Many people grew up in homes that were very dysfunctional; where they experienced mental, physical and verbal abuse, lack and poverty, and instability. And some have grown up in an environment where one or both of the parents were drinkers, or drug abuser, and have had to experience them mentally, and physically abusing one another. As a child it is not easy watching someone you love go through such abuse, and it not only affects you while it is happening, but will also affect you for many years down the line. There are actually people who were affected to the degree that, it was many years after a particular person passed away before they were able to forgive them, and receive healing from the pain associated with what they've experienced.

What people experience in the home while growing up can also have an effect on their marriage in the sense that, it could cause you to go into a relationship always seeing the bad traits of your father in your husband, and it can also cause you to see the bad traits of your mother when it comes to your wife. If for example you didn't have a good relationship with your father and you are a female, you may subconsciously find yourself looking for the father figure that you never had. And therefore when choosing a mate instead of looking for the characteristics that you should want in a husband, you are really looking for the characteristics that were lacking in your father. Because of this you could wind up marrying someone much older than yourself, and as the two of you grow older, this age gap may cause problems for the marriage.

The mind can be very fragile therefore you must protect it. We have all had many different experiences, both good and bad. Some have seemingly left us scarred for life, and as much as we might like to eliminate our unhealthy thoughts that have come as a result of these experiences, it's not easy. This is because the negative thoughts have been integrated with the thoughts we want to retain, by way of the subconscious, conscious, and unconscious parts of the mind. The mind is the center of consciousness that not only generates thoughts, feelings, ideas, and perceptions, but also records and stores memories that consists of accumulative information. This information includes the thoughts, conclusions, decisions, observations, and perceptions of the person their self throughout their entire existence. In other words, everything that we have ever done, thought, observed, experienced or perceived have been recorded, and things that we thought we had forgotten are still stored in our mind.

Whether we realize it or not every negative experience we encounter will help to shape our lives. They can distort the way we think; corrupting our mind, and keeping us from moving forward in life. Many people today are still stuck in their childhood, because they haven't been able to move past the point of an experience that has devastated them. It is said that if a child grows up in the home of an alcoholic that there's a good chance that they'll also become an alcoholic, or if a child grows up in an abusive home there's a good chance that they'll become abusive. And just as they watched their father for example physically abuse their mother, they too will do the same thing to their wife. This doesn't necessarily mean he doesn't love her, but because he grew up watching this type of behavior in my father, it affected how he dealt with situations in his own marriage. This type of negative influence is very similar to what is known as suggestive thoughts. They are thoughts that can enter the mind through a leading, an enticement, a proposition, or by one alluding to something, they are also ideas or images that are formed in the mind as a result of something that has been said or done.

Every person in this world has been or will be influenced at one point or another by a suggestive thought, whether it is deliberate or not. There is no way around it, because we are constantly being introduced to these ideas or images no matter where we are or what we're doing, whether it is via conversation, what we see or read, or what we hear on television or the radio. Oftentimes there are people that influence our lives and even the decisions we make without ever realizing it, and some of these influences are good and some are bad. The most commonly used category for suggestive thoughts are those that are rude or improper, especially those of a sexual nature, however not all suggestive thoughts come in a negative form. There are those who genuinely care about us, and will also put thoughts in our mind through an association of different ideas by saying things like; why don't you eat better? Take better care of yourself, quit smoking, or you need to lose weight. These ideas once spoken will enter the heart, and may incite a person to do very positive things that will benefit them greatly, but usually the greater affect is brought on by the more negative suggestions.

Children who grow up in inner city neighborhoods live challenged lives, and often become a by-product of the type of atmosphere or surroundings they were forced to live in. why? Because the images of these surroundings that were placed in their minds as children as misguiding as they were, spoke volumes to them as to how life is supposed to be. For example; they can leave them with thoughts such as, I have no choice but to do this to survive. I'm not worthy of anything better. They don't have anything so why would I? and the list goes on. Unfortunately, many of them grow up and embark on a journey that leads to a life that is full of crime and abuse, which ultimately lands them either in prison or the grave. Although this is more noticeable in areas where financially challenged families live. Pain does not discriminate and there are many people throughout the world who have been exposed to negative suggestions. Some of them are wealthy, some have great careers, wonderful families, are part of the corporate world, and are very successful in what they do. However, because of the thoughts they were exposed to they still struggle nonetheless because of the negative influence.

Many people are silently hurting as a result of things they had to endure throughout life. Because they are ashamed to let anyone know what they've been through, they go through life dealing with hurt and suffering alone. To look at some of them you would never know that they were suffering, because people have become very good at masking their problems, but if you could take a look inside their mind you would see the pain. And you would also find that we live in a world full of people who just like you, and me are in need of help, and who also have a story to tell. It may not be the same as your story, but it's just as important to them as yours is to you. Suggestive thoughts affect everyone, it doesn't matter what your race, size, status, or gender is. It doesn't matter whether you're saved or unsaved. No one is exempt. Although we fall prey to these sorts of thoughts as children we don't have to remain in bondage to them or their offspring. The offspring of suggestive thoughts are the active results we have to deal with on a daily basis, such as complications or problems, improper mindsets, erroneous lifestyles, and pain and suffering.

What you need to understand is that pain and brokenness usually doesn't start when you reach adulthood, but rather it starts when you are a child and, you are first introduced to negative situations, negative surroundings and negative relationships. These things have been embedded in your heart and mind in the early stages of life when you were very vulnerable, and impressionable and is allowed to lie within you, festering for many years. By the time you realize there's a problem, and when and where it began, and then take the steps necessary to make a diagnosis and bring healing to the situation, it can be like trying to unravel the most intricate web, and it's very difficult to determine where to begin. Many people will never share their painful experiences with others because of shame, and trust issues. There are others who don't have an understanding of how to process what they've experienced, and become very frustrated at the thought of talking about it, so they hold it in and deal with it the best that they know how to. However, they still need help understanding when the pain began, and where it originated.

This is very important, because until you do this you will never be able to find a starting point, where you can begin to dissect what you're feeling, or what you're dealing with, and this is essential if you are to ever sort out your issues and come to a place of healing. Healing is essential because without it, just as physical pain has the ability to affect your entire body, emotional pain has the ability to affect your entire life, and because of it, many people are likely to die on the inside long before their physical body ever does.

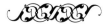

CHAPTER 2

Understanding the Complexity of the Heart

THE HEART CAN be very tricky in the sense that if you allow it to it will take you down a winding path, and steer you in a direction that you never wanted to take.

The heart is the center of one's emotions; the place that your emotions occupy and from which they originate. It is the place where your thoughts, will, and decisions originate and proceed out of. The condition of your heart determines whether or not you are able to give, and receive love, compassion or affection.

Your heart is the core of your being or the central area that houses everything which determines who you are, such as your personality, disposition, character and nature. It contains one's emotions, deals with feelings such as anger, bitterness, rage, joy, happiness, loneliness, etc. Imagine having one central area where all of these different feelings are constantly flowing back and forth. The emotions that we display depends upon what happens to us from moment to moment, and from day to day; like how others treat us, how we feel physically, what kind of stress we deal with at work or at home, and what someone says to us.

There are many people whose emotions are literally all over the place. One moment they're glad, and then they're mad. Today they're happy, and tomorrow they're sad. This is because they are not emotionally stable. The definition for stable is that which is not likely to move, not readily undergoing change, constant, and unwavering. In others words when something is stable It doesn't sway back and forth. It's not up and down, in and out and all over the place. But when you allow your emotions to get out of control, this is ultimately what happens. You wind up being tossed to and fro by everything that happens, and by everything someone says or does. So what I am saying is that you must learn how to bring your emotions under control and not allow them to control you.

Whether you realize it or not, the heart and the mind are connected. As I said in chapter one, the mind is the center of consciousness that generates thoughts, feelings, ideas, and perceptions, and also records and stores memories through a collection of information. The heart is the place that your emotions occupy, and where your thoughts, will, and decisions originate. As we take in information whether it is via conversation, things we see on television, hear on the radio, read in a book, or something that happens to us or around us, this information then enters the heart. Although you may think the mind is where you meditate or think about the information you take in it's not. The heart is where we ponder the information or think about it.

Many times you you'll hear someone talking about pondering things in the heart, but not the mind. The definition for ponder is to consider carefully, and some of the synonyms for it is to think about, contemplate, deliberate, or meditate upon. So your thoughts actually originate in the heart, not the mind. Now remember, the heart is where your emotions are located, so depending on what information you take in, this will determine which of your emotions are activated, and that emotion will then determine which decisions you make, and the actions you take. So as you ponder a thought, in your heart it is then transferred to the mind where the memories of these events are stored. The mind has the ability to generate thoughts, feelings, ideas, and perceptions, but all of these things originate from the heart as the information that we take in sparks our emotions.

This is why it is so important to be careful of what information we take into our eye gates and our ear gates.

In dealing with the heart, sense it is where your thoughts, will, and decisions originate you must be careful to keep it as healthy as possible. As you enter into relationships with people, you actually enter into their world. As you begin to care for these people, their problems will become your problems. Their pain can affect you, and so can their unhealthy habits. Anything negative that happens as a result of you venturing off into someone else's world can affect the wellbeing of your heart. When you have minimal contact with other people, you can pretty much control what happens in your life, and even the problems you have will be very limited. Keep in mind though, that while it may sound like a quick way to solve this type of issue, it would not be advisable for you to cut yourself off from other people, because this too can be unhealthy. But it is a fact that when you open yourself up to others you can become vulnerable, and you can then be subjected to things that would make for an unhealthy heart. An unhealthy heart is one that has been injured through loss. It is also one that has been injured by way of being deceived and taken advantage of, mental and physical abuse, rejection, abandonment and a host of other things. Therefore, you must be careful who you trust with your heart, and who you allow to become a part of your life.

Everyone has hopes and dreams, and many have had promises made to them, but many years can go by without ever seeing those hopes and dreams or the promises come into manifestation. Because the heart is the seat of the emotions, as time passes and none of these things take place, you can feel as if you're at a standstill, and that your life is slipping away. It is also at this point that emotions are stirred up, and you may begin to wonder whether or not everything you've done have been done in vain, whether or not your time will ever come, and why things never work out for you. You may also begin to challenge your choices, feeling as though you will never get ahead, never get married, if that is one of your desires and that you'll never be happy. As these things are pondered in the heart they will begin to wear on it. You become tired, sad, and, weary and if you're not careful this is where you will begin to lose hope. If you believe in God, and you know what His word says and you've received a word of prophesy from Him, and you know that you have done everything you're supposed to do, but you don't see anything manifest over a long period of time, this can be very disappointing and damaging to the heart as well. However, as you begin to see your hopes, dreams, and promises come into fruition it can cause a wellspring of joy to fill up inside of you, strengthening the heart, making it happy, and bringing life and health to it.

The heart just like the mind can be very fragile, and many times you will be accused of being overly sensitive about certain things. In some cases, this can be true, but in most cases it is simply that, the heart can become so overloaded with so many things at one time, that it will begin to work overtime trying to process everything, and this can cause your emotions to be all over the place. Sometimes you feel angry, the next moment you feel sad and out of nowhere you want to cry. You feel a tinge of joy, and then all of a sudden confusion sets in and you're trying to make sense of all of this while feeling like you're on a rollercoaster ride that you want to get off of, but it just keeps going around and around.

Some people have been through a lot more than others and can have years and years of unpleasant memories stored in the mind. If you're not careful you will take these mental notes out of storage and begin to ponder them in your heart all over again. The problem with this is that as you experience things, they are stored in the mind one by one, however as you begin to look at these things again you don't just open one mental note and put it back, and then open another one. You open one and set it aside, and then open another one and set it aside, and before you know it you have all of this baggage open and now you're looking at all of it at the same time. All of those memories are flooding your heart, and now you've gotten all of these different emotions stirred up all over again and this can become very overwhelming. When you find yourself in a situation like this it may be to your benefit, to find someone to talk to who can help you sort all of these things out one by one so that you can get rid of them.

Scripture have given us a clear description of the heart of an un-regenerated or unsaved person. This is a heart that has not been changed, and still has all of the character traits of the old nature that comes from Adam. It's full of deception, there is nothing you can do to fix it, and because it is so complex you will never be able to understand all of the internal workings of it. You hear people saying all of the time that you should follow your heart, but if you're honest with yourself, you will admit that much of the trouble you get into is because you do allow yourself to be led by your heart.

When you've been hurt so badly some many times it is a natural reaction to want to shut your heart, and not allow anyone else to have access to it, because you're thinking if you don't let yourself get close to anyone else you won't get hurt anymore. This is the only way that you can think of to protect yourself and it's perfectly understandable. The problem with this is that at some point you could find yourself becoming shut off from the world. You'll find yourself missing out on a lot of healthy relationships that you could otherwise have, and if you're not careful you will allow your heart to trick you out of something that is good for you.

No one knows for sure what will happen to him or her, if anything will happen at all or for that matter when it will happen. Your heart will convince you based upon your past experiences, that everyone you enter into a relationship with is going to hurt you, and that you'll be better off by yourself. It can also convince you that you're going to die at a certain age of a specific illness or disease, because other men or women in your family died of the same thing at the same age. Fear is one of the emotions that occupy your heart. This emotion works hand in hand with doubt and will cause you to become stagnated, keep you from moving forward and rob you of your happiness.

It vital that you pay close attention to what you have read in this chapter, so that you can gain an understanding of the condition of your heart, why it is in this condition and how you can avoid any further damage to it. You also need to have an understanding of the type of affects that it can, and will have on your life if you allow your emotions to go unchecked and get out of control. It was never meant for your emotions to control you, but rather you are supposed to have control over them. Remember, your heart is the place that your emotions occupy, and the place that your will, your thoughts, and your decisions originate. If you do not have control of that which occupies your heart, then you will forever lack the ability to make the correct decisions for your life. In addition, you will have no control over the thoughts or the decisions that you do make, because you will continue to do everything based upon your painful past experiences, forever looking behind you and allowing your past to keep you paralyzed by the fear of what has happened, therefore giving it the power to determine the timing and the course of your future.

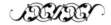

CHAPTER 3

You Are Not Alone

IF IT WERE meant for us to be alone in the world there would've been no need for the earth to be populated, and in order for us to go through this life successfully, we must connect with people. As we go through life we meet many different people, and have the ability and the right to pick and choose which of those people we want to be a part of our life. As stated in chapter two, as we enter into relationships we enter into that person's world, so along with the person and the relationship comes many different situations and circumstances, both good and bad. Everyone wants to love and be loved whether they admit it or not, and one of the scariest things in life is the feeling of being all alone, having no one to and share your life with. We live in a society where abandonment seems to be very prevalent, relationships don't seem to be a priority anymore and people walk away from them just as easily as they change their clothing. Commitment seems to be a thing of the past, and people do not believe it is important to keep their word on any level. Most households today only have one parent and the statistics are quite staggering. According to statistics a total of 15 million children in America are being raised without a father, another 5 million are being raised without a mother, and about 50% of all marriages in America end in divorce.

Even though both adults and children are abandoned it usually has a greater effect on children, and this is a very serious issue. Each parent has a role that is vital to a child. A mother can't teach her son how to be a man, and a father can't teacher his daughter how to be a woman. On the flip side the son needs his mother to cover, and nurture him and teach him, and a daughter need her father to love and protect her. Whenever one of the two is missing, so is a part of what each child needs. Even if the child never knew the parent that is missing they will still feel a sense of abandonment. For those who have two parents, but lose one due to divorce they not only feel a sense of abandonment, but many times they will grow up blaming their self for the break-up of their parents. This weighs very heavily on children even to the point of causing them to have a condition called "Abandoned Child Syndrome." This is a behavioral or psychological condition that result from the loss of one or both parents. Abandonment experiences are never the fault of the child, yet the wounds are seated deep within their young hearts and minds. The pain is very real to them and can be felt throughout their life, becoming a driving force long after they become adults, and in order for this condition to be reversed they need to be able to both accept and understand the cause of the injury. Because of abandonment many children grow up feeling as if they are all alone in the world, even though they are surrounded by a host of people who love them.

Those who have been in relationships where their spouse or partner walked out on them, this act of abandonment still has the ability to cause deep pain, and will still have a lasting affect on their life as well. It is also a fact that one doesn't have to be absent from a person's life in order to abandon them, and in fact they can actually be right in the same household. One of the most common affects abandonment has on both children and adults is that they develop trust issues. When someone makes a commitment to love you and be a part of your life and then leaves you, it can take a very long time for you to trust the commitment of another person. This is one of the most common causes of people holding on to baggage throughout their life and taking it into other relationships. When people are abandoned they will begin to not only have trust issues, but also insecurities. Some will blame themselves and others will blame everyone else that they come into relationship with. You must keep in mind that usually the root of your pain doesn't begin when you become an adult, but it most likely started when you were a child. In some cases, when a child deals with abandonment if you watch them close enough, you will see that long after they become an adult, in many ways they are still in that child's mind, desiring to be loved, and wanted by the person that abandoned them, and continuously striving to win that person's approval. As a result of this and a host of other experiences many people live in their own private hell. They are unwilling to trust for fear that they will be let down again, believing they are all alone in what they're going through, that no one cares and that no one understands, so they hold on to their pain and dare not share what they're feeling. When you watch someone that is very dear to your heart suffer from this very thing for many years, it makes you wish you could go back into the past and change things, to prevent the pain and suffering that has taken place in their life as a result of this abandonment.

The phrase "hurting people hurt people" makes so much sense. This is so true, and is the main reason why there are so many hurting people in the world today. It is the people who are hurting that is most likely to hurt someone else and especially the ones they love. Many times they may not even realize what they're doing and why they're doing it, and in some cases many don't know how to stop. Sometimes they hurt those they love not because it's something that they've set out to do, but because in many cases they're just acting out what they saw in their home, or what took place in the environment that they grew up in. When someone hurts you there is a possibility that for many years after that person is deceased, you may still struggle with the pain of what you've experienced. Generally, when we get hurt, because we are in the midst of our own pain, it is never taken into consideration what kind of pain that person may have been carrying around all of those years that may have eventually led to them hurting us. We usually never think about what kind of childhood they may have had, or what kind of environment they may have grown up in. And it's so crazy how things that happen in our lives can have such a rippling affect, and how we can actually be a repeat of someone else and what they have done to us.

I'm pleading with you to break the cycle today. You don't have to continue to live this way. You are not alone, and you can prevent yourself from continuing to be a victim of your past environment, and the pain that you've experienced at the hand of someone else that may have been hurting too, and if you have children you can also prevent them from becoming a victim of pain and abandonment, and from repeating the same cycle all over again.

When you experience things like abandonment, and rejection as adults you may deal with it differently than a child, but the experience is just as painful, and the pain is still just as real. I've never heard of an abandoned adult syndrome, however the damage still needs to be reversed and if this is going to happen, just as with children, the issues must be dealt with. Abandonment can have many different affects on the life of an adult. In many cases it can cause you to question your self-worth. When entering relationships, if you find someone who might be a good partner, you will begin looking for their faults, and instead of looking for what is right with them you begin looking for what's wrong. The thought of being alone and going through life's difficulties by yourself can be overwhelming, yet you find yourself withdrawing from other people.

When experiencing trauma, it can have a lasting effect, which can cause you to go into a shell and clam up, because although you may have a fear of being alone, your fear of trusting again is even greater and you will wind up pushing away anyone that you feel would potentially hurt you. When you continue to focus on past experiences you can quickly find yourself stuck somewhere between your past and your future never able to go any further. It's like driving a car, and even though your goal is to move forward, because you spend so much time looking in the rearview mirror, it becomes an interference that obstructs your view, making your journey impossible. When trying to drive forward while looking through the rearview mirror, your sight will always be limited, and you will never get very far, because you can't look behind you and in front of yourself at the same time.

The bigger picture is always in front of you, and as you move forward it becomes clearer, and the greater your odds of obtaining your dreams and aspirations become. It is not a coincidence that as you move forward you get closer to where you want to go, and further away from that which is behind you. There are many things that you will pass along the road of life, and if you allow it to, it will hold you back, but you must determine which is more important. Is it that which you are moving towards or that which you are moving away from? You cannot have both any more than you can move in both directions at the same time. Just as surely as this is true, it is also true that you can't live in your past and your future at the same time. You only have two hands and therefore, in life if you cannot continue to hold on to the things of the past, and expect to be able to grab a hold of the future that awaits you. Your past was only meant to serve as a tool to teach, strengthen, and prepare you for the fulfillment of the purpose for which you were born.

Don't allow your past experiences no matter how painful, to hold you hostage and put you in solitary confinement. Just as there is evil in this world, there is also good. It would be wonderful if we knew in advance what was going to happen to us at every turn, but unfortunately that's not the way it works. Our journey in life can at times be like opening a box of cracker jacks. As you open each box there is a different prize, and though you didn't know what you would receive, as a kid you were full of excitement and anticipation at the thought of opening that box and finding out what your prize would be. Life is far greater than a box of caramel corn and some peanuts, and the blessings that await you are far greater than a plastic ring or some other toy. So dare to step out and take a chance at life. Learn how to trust again and defy the odds of abandonment and everything else that would try and convince you that nobody cares, and nobody wants you. You are very important, very much needed, very much wanted and you are not alone.

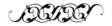

CHAPTER 4

Unmasking the Pain

FEAR IS SOMETHING that many of us struggle with on a daily basis. One of the definitions of fear is an unpleasant feeling of anxiety or apprehension, caused by the presence or anticipation of danger. It is also said to be "False Evidence Appearing Real." The struggle with fear is something that is very real for many people. Many times because of their inability to deal with certain situations, and their own personal struggle with how they think people will perceive them, people have been known to draw a picture in their mind of what they believe something to be, even though the opposite is true. At times no matter how much someone tries to convince them that what they believe is incorrect, because of their own insecurities, they are unable to accept what is said as truth. They dig up false evidence that they have created or generated through information that they have fed into their own mind, and then convince themselves that it is real. Because of this many struggle with the fear of success, the fear of the unknown, the fear of failure, the fear of lack, the fear of loss, and etc., but one of the things that is becoming more prevalent throughout society is the fear of revealing to others that we are in pain.

For whatever reason people tend to think that if someone sees that they're in pain, they will somehow view them as being weak, and they're ashamed to let it be known that they were at some point vulnerable, as if this somehow makes them less than a man or a woman. They fear others finding out that they're in trouble. This has more to do with pride than anything else, and is usually true more so with men than it is with women. It is sometimes hard to admit that they've allowed themselves to be open enough for someone or something to hurt them. They don't want anyone to pity them, and don't want to appear as if they stand in need of help, so they'll put on a mask and pretend that everything is okay. Pain, just like offenses, is something that is inevitable. It is something that we will never be able to totally avoid, and just as sure as we live we are all going to experience some form of pain in this life.

A mask is a façade, a disguise, or a face covering used to hide one's identity. So when someone puts on a mask they are trying to conceal something. However, masks were never meant for permanent use. As it is stated in chapter one there are many people in this world who are in pain, and who walk around suffering greatly on a daily basis, but because they have had so much practice disguising their pain you would never be able to look at them and know they were hurting. Normally the setting in which you would see a mask is at a masquerade ball, as you know, this is a place where everyone who attends comes dressed up as someone that they are not, because the whole point is to pretend to be someone you're not. But they go beyond just putting on a mask. They must also dress the part. So they put on wigs, mustaches, glasses and clothing to make this illusion of who they are pretending to be seem real. There is a song that goes like this; "the whole world is a stage and everybody's playing a part." As we go through life masking our pain we too are acting out a role, playing a part and pretending to be something that we are not. The only difference is that we don't put on costumes instead we put on smiles, pretending to be happy when we're really sad, and laughing when we really want to cry.

As we go through various trials and tribulations in life, though we are able to endure the experiences, it will be beneficial for others if we share with them what we have been through and how we were able to actually make it through and survive. In other words, the very fact that someone else was able to go through what they were suffering and come out unscathed and with their mind still intact will give them hope that they too will be able to survive. Many of us while we are ashamed to share what we have come through are really just depriving the next person of some very vital information that will serve to strengthen them, give them hope and help build up their faith. In a court of law, a testimony is proof, evidence, verification, and a statement of the fact. And as we share our testimony it basically says hey, you know what? This experience didn't kill me, and I am living proof that it will not kill you either. I made it through this storm, and I'm still standing. I still have my sanity, and my health has also remained intact, therefore I am living proof for you that it can be done, and that you will be able to overcome this obstacle also. If you pay attention to the word testimony you will notice that the first four letters spell out the word test. A test is something that is difficult. It is a painful situation, or somebody or something troublesome and without the test there is no testimony. Notice that in each of these definitions some form of pain is present, and therefore is a mandatory part of the test. A testimony is therefore proof, evidence, a verification of and a witness to the fact that you are capable of both enduring, and overcoming many painful experiences. Your testimony is not for you, it is for those who are going through the same or similar tests, and who need to know that though it may appear as if it is going to get the best of them, someone has proven that it's possible to overcome even the most difficult obstacles. And while it is very tempting to hold on to your evidence or statement of facts, you must share it otherwise it does you no good to have gone through it all.

Masking your pain is equivalent to putting a band aide on a wound that is in need of stitches. No matter how many you apply, because the root cause of the issue has not been dealt with it will only grow worse. You can only smile your way through your pain and pretend it doesn't exist for so long. Pain is just like steam, you may be able to hold it in and cover it up for a long period of time, but the pressure just keeps building, and building and in the long run you wind up doing yourself more harm than good. As you mask your pain and go about your life pretending that it doesn't exist, just as surely as you live, you are going to run into other obstacles in your journey through life that will also be painful. The more you endure, the more you hold in, and the more you hold in the more build up you will have. Steam can only build up for so long before it has to be released. As it builds it will outgrow the space in which it is confined, and as this happens it builds up what is called combustion. Combustion is a chemical reaction, ignition, or an extreme agitation. When it builds up to a certain point it must be released, and usually when it reaches this point there is going to be an explosion of some sort. The size of the explosion will depend largely upon how much of a buildup there is. As you allow your pain to build up one day your heart and your mind is going to go into overload. A form of combustion due to the stress, and strain of life, all of the painful experiences, and everything else you've been dealing with is going to overwhelm you and all of a sudden without warning everything inside of you will come out all at once.

My advice to you is this; stop masking your pain. It is not healthy for you on a mental or a physical level. It is okay to let other people know that you are human. I'll let you in on a little secret, they already know, and usually your perception of what you appear to be is different from everyone else's anyway. While it is important how others see us, it is even more important how we see ourselves. We are usually our worst critics, and sometimes we are just too hard on our self. We all have strengths and weaknesses. It is one of the things that make us who we are. Pain is something that we all experience whether we like it or not, and no one is exempt. It is absolutely okay to say hey, I'm in trouble or hey I'm hurting. If you don't feel comfortable talking with family or friends there are many people who get paid to listen to all of your problems, and who also have the ability to help you take those things that you don't know what to do with and sort them out. Masks were made for temporary use. They were not made for the heart but for the face, and stress will kill you one way or another if you allow it to. You may not have any control over your past experiences, and whether or not you become a victim of certain circumstances, but you do have control over whether or not you remain a victim. So guess what? The masquerade is over, and it's time to take off the mask.

If you desire to be healed from the pain and brokenness you feel, the first step is to take the mask off and stop pretending that everything is okay. This is absolutely necessary. Whether you're dealing with drugs, alcohol, gambling, sex, fear, or anything else, the first step is to acknowledge that you have a problem. Until you take this first step you will never be set free. The pain that has you bound is not the problem. The problem is the thing that you have experienced, and that you must deal with and move past. No one wakes up one day and says you know what? I'm in pain, but nothing has happened for me to be in pain, I'm just hurting. No, there has to be a root cause for any pain that you are dealing with. It doesn't matter whether the pain is physical or emotional something has happened to cause this pain. And the reason why it is so hard for us to sometimes move past it is because we don't want to disclose that which we have experienced. We don't want to say, you know what? Yes, I am hurting, and this is why, but this is the key to getting healed and moving forward. You must deal with the root cause and there is no way around it.

Depending upon the depth of the trauma that you've experienced you may eventually find yourself convinced, that if you don't talk about it you won't have to deal with it, and it will eventually go away. But just because you don't talk about something, that doesn't mean it will go away. In fact, if you don't talk about it and get the load off of your heart, it will never go away, but will probably get worse. Do you know why? Let's go back to chapter two. Remember, everything that you have experienced throughout your life has been recorded and stored in your mind, and whether you want it to or not, occasionally those memories will be triggered through conversation, something you see, and even certain places that you go. The memory of that experience will never be wiped from your mind, and depending on how deep the trauma was, and how deeply rooted the pain is, it can and will haunt you for the rest of your life. In many cases this can cause you to wind up going into a place of seclusion, convinced that if you build a wall around yourself no one will ever be able to hurt you again. If you are not careful it is very possible that you will fall off into a depression, have a mental melt down of some sort, and eventually get to a point where no one is able to reach you. Worse than this, even though the mask you wear may seem to be convenient, and it seems to be serving the purpose for which you bought it, and though you might feel comfortable wearing it, someday you could very well look into a mirror, and find that because you have been wearing it for so long, not only have you come to a place where you have become unrecognizable to others, but you have also come to a place where you no longer recognize yourself.

Do yourself a favor and unmask your pain before it's too late. Don't be like the person who was on fire and because they saw the smoke but didn't see any flames, instead of taking action while they still had time they decided to fan the smoke in an effort to make it go away. They didn't realize that smoke is usually the first sign that a fire is in progress, and while they were fanning the flames they were really contributing the wind that was necessary for the fire to spread and the rest is history.

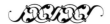

CHAPTER 5

Pushing Past the Pain

IN THIS CHAPTER you will learn the art of identifying and pushing past the obstacles that stand in front of you. An obstacle is something in the way, and is synonymous of an obstruction, or a stumbling block. When something obstructs your view, it can limit what you see, therefore interfering with your ability to see something for what it really is, or it blocks your view altogether, leaving you totally unaware of what lies ahead. A stumbling block stands in the way of achieving a goal, and is a difficulty that causes mistakes or prevents progress. In this instance the obstacle seems to be the pain, but even though the pain is very significant and seems to be the main focus of what stands in your way, there are other components that when combined together, is actually the foundation that the pain is built upon. So pain is the offspring or the end result of something far greater, which is the foundation or the primary cause of the pain. So when you're dealing with an obstacle which has the ability to limit or block your view of something, it can at the same time cause you to make mistakes and ultimately prevent your progress, and therefore keep you from moving forward.

Of the two emotions, which is pain and joy, if you were to experience both of them simultaneously, and to a very high degree, the one that would affect you the most and therefore occupy more of your time would be pain. This is the case not just because painful experiences have the ability to arouse so many different emotions consecutively, but because the emotions that are often awakened by pain, such as anger, rage, bitterness, hatred, and sadness are usually some of the more dominant emotions. Because of this when you deal with a great degree of pain it has the ability to obstruct your view, and can easily be confused as the obstacle that you need to push past, but it's not. Yes, you need to be able to push past your pain however it will not take place the way you think it will, and this is because, as I said before, your pain is merely the end result of the experience that have taken place. In order to push past your pain, you must be willing to deal with all of the issues, which is the foundation that the pain was built upon.

When building a home there must first be a foundation, because without a foundation, you basically have nowhere to start, so the first thing that takes place after surveying the land is the excavation or digging of a hole. Once the excavation is completed and most of the technical work is done, the foundation is then constructed by pouring concrete, determining the proper thickness of the foundation walls and then allowing it to properly set. There are many different components that goes into laying the foundation of a home, and if you wanted to tear that house down and build a different one in its place, because the structure of a foundation for each house is different, in order for you to move forward and build again in that spot you would have to deal with removing each piece of the foundation. Likewise, the foundation of your pain starts with a deep hole that has been dug in your heart, and is comprised of the many experiences you've had to endure, such as abandonment, rejection, mental and physical abuse, rape, incest, adultery, being lied on, deceived and etc. and must be dealt with one component at a time, if you ever expect to push past your pain and begin to rebuild your life. One of the key differences between the foundation of your pain, and that of a house is that, once you dig the hole for a foundation of a home, and the concrete is poured and set, that hole will never go any deeper than what it is at that point and time, because everything is already set in place. But as time goes by, and you have more and more painful experiences, the hole that has being dug in your heart has no set depth, and can continue to go deeper and deeper, doing an insurmountable amount of damage and could potentially ruin your life.

When you have an obstacle that is blocking your path, you have no choice but to move it if you plan to go forward, and the only real way to do that, is to find the weakest points, where there is less weight, and begin pushing. Pushing requires Perseverance, understanding, strength and heart, but when pushing past the obstacles you have to remember, that you're not just pushing past what see, but you're actually pushing past all of the hidden things; those issues that caused the pain in the first place, and this is why this obstacle is so heavy and so hard to move. For example; your pain may be the overall obstacle that you need to push past, but the things that have caused you so much pain is what torments you on a daily basis. This is because as you sit and ponder the memories of each painful event that's been recorded and stored in your mind, the hurt that you feel is like having a deep cut, and each time it grows a scab you sit and pick at it, and pull it off. So the bleeding starts all over again, but so does the pain, and as a matter of fact each time the scab is pulled off the wound becomes more and more, irritated and the pain feels just as fresh and just as bad as it did the day you were injured.

This is also true for your heart. The healing process for your heart begins, but as you ponder the painful memories of yesterday, you wind up pulling the scab off of those old wounds. But the difference between a cut and the heart, is that the wounds in the heart are usually a lot deeper than they seem, and the scars that you have are mental scars. So as you pull the scabs off, your mind immediately takes you right back to the very moment that the event took place, and the pain becomes just as fresh as the day it happened. The problem with that is this, when dealing with a cut it's generally just one cut and therefore one scab, so even though it hurts the pain is compartmentalized, and confined to one specific location and after a little while it will subside. But when dealing with the heart there are many wounds and therefore many scabs, and as you begin to ponder those memories you don't just stop at one event, but it becomes much like a rippling effect, and you move on from one to the next, and then the next, and so on and so forth. Before you know it you have all of these memories flooding your mind at one time and can see no end of the pain in sight.

Pain seems to be the overall obstacle that you're dealing with because it has been allowed to build up so much over a long period of time, but it only exists because of all of your traumatic past experiences. In many cases it will take a toll on every area of your life; affecting your health, your appetite, and whether or not you sleep. It will hinder your desire to socialize with other people, and sometimes even your ability to go to work or carry on with the normal functions of life. In other words, it can, and will totally consume you if you allow it to.

In order to push past the pain, you must first determine its source, in other words, what was the root cause of the pain? Once you determine that you will have to deal with the root of each individual issue. Issues are much like weeds. You never know when or where they might spring up, both of them can grow while unattended, and they also grow under the most severe conditions. In addition to this, just as with weeds, when attempting to get rid of an issue, if you only deal with it on the surface it may appear to be gone, but will surely resurface. When dealing with any issue you cannot just ignore the root, and then expect for it to go away. The root is the life of the issue just as it is the life of a plant, and unless you destroy the root you will forever have to face the issue, and this is what happens to many individuals.

Depending on the situation you are dealing with, it can be a very tough ordeal when it comes to sorting out and addressing all of the painful details. This is especially so in cases of rape, incest, or abuse of any kind. Many women who have been raped would rather let it go and try to live with what has happened to them, rather than face their attacker in the court room where they will be subjected to the questions of the defense attorney, and the embarrassment and humiliation of giving a bunch of complete strangers a full account of what has happened. It's too much like reliving the act all over again. So for some people it's just easier to skip over certain issues and not deal with them at all. The problem with that is this, in ignoring the situation and choosing not to deal with it, you are giving your pain permission to stick around and plague you for the rest of your life.

You must make a choice, and in doing this you must ask yourself if you would rather deal with the pain of facing your issues head on once and for all, knowing that at the end of the day you will be rid of the pain, and agony forever, or if you would rather keep all of these things bottled up inside of you, continue to live a life of constant pain and torment and become a shell of a person while slowly dying on the inside. I strongly encourage you to face your problems and deal with them, and remember, you don't have to deal with all of your issues at one time, it's easier to push past the obstacle in front of you when you find and deal with the weakest points first. The weakest point of the obstacle for you might be that someone that you trusted lied to you or used you. Once you deal with those areas and get rid of some of the weight that has been holding you down, then you will have more strength to push past the tougher or heavier issues. This might be scary, and it might not be the easiest thing you've ever done, but it's a process and every process consists of a series of steps, but just as it is with walking, every time you take a step you move forward and push past the pain of different obstacles. Before you know it you will get up one day and find that there is nothing holding you back any longer and now you are free to move on and enjoy the rest of your life.

Many times the mere thought of dealing with certain situations can be scary, and exhausting and this makes you want to give up before you even get started. You must make a conscience decision and an effort to take back your life and move forward, but this starts by facing your past head on and making the decision that what has happened to you will no longer control your life. The only way anything or anyone can have the opportunity to control you is if you first relinquish your control. Greatness stands in front of you and the only way that you will ever receive it is to reach out and grab hold of it. Yes, you're tired, I get it, but your future is worth fighting for and you have to want it bad enough, and then you must believe it. It's so easy to just give up, but that is the coward's way out and you are anything but a coward. Just because someone hits you, and knocks you down it doesn't mean you have to stay there.

This is going to sound crazy, but did you know it is possible to make pain your friend? Whenever you are faced with a situation how you deal with it all depends upon how you view it. If you never experience anything you will never learn anything, and if you never learn anything you will forever remain the same. Is it fun getting hurt? No, but check this out. When a person decides that they want to become a boxer for example, long before they ever step into the ring to have that initial fight, they know that they must go through a stage of training and preparation. This training and preparation consists of grueling exercise to build stamina, muscle training or bodybuilding and also sparring. This goes on for months and sometimes years, and all of this takes place long before they ever get the opportunity to get in the ring and have their first fight. They are fully aware of the fact that this time of training and preparation is going to be painful, and there will probably be many times that they will want to give up, but they refuse to because they are also aware of the fact that, as painful as it may be they know three things and that is this. It's what they want, it's worth it, and once the initial training is over, even though they will have to continue training throughout their career to stay in shape, the worst part is over. Now here's the key. Everything they went through was very painful, but it was also very necessary and at the end of the day everything they had to endure made them stronger, not weaker.

The trials and tribulations we endure are meant to make us strong not weak, but will make us weak if we continue to look at them in a negative manner, and allow them to suck all of the energy out of us. Just as the boxer builds strength and stamina as they endure pain, as we go through trials and tribulations we are supposed to gain strength and stamina as well. Each painful experience that we go through strengthens and prepares us for what is to come next. Anything that does not kill you should make you stronger, and if you look at your painful experiences in this light, you will find in the long run that pain really isn't the enemy that you thought it was, but instead it is really your friend. Some of the things you are going through right now at this very moment would kill you if it hadn't been for the things that you've already gone through, because what you're going through right now is so painful that there is no way you could have survived it if the other experiences hadn't come along and helped to build you up and give you the strength to be able to handle it. So instead of despising what you have been through learn to embrace it, because as painful as it may have been it really did serve a purpose, and a very vital one at that. So push past your pain with the thought that, the obstacle that is standing in front of you doesn't really have control over you, but instead you have control over it. And as you push forward no matter how hard it may seem, continue to say to yourself, I can, I must, and I will.

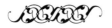

CHAPTER 6

Identifying the Source of Your Pain

AS EXPLAINED IN chapter 4, the only way you will ever be able to move past your emotional pain and heal is to understand that though the pain you feel seems to be the overall obstacle that keeps you from moving forward, it is really just the offspring of a traumatic event. The true obstacle is the issues that resulted in the pain you're experiencing, but you cannot see this because of the obstruction that is blocking your view, and the most efficient way to remove this obstacle is to find its weakest points meaning your smaller issues, and deal with them first. In doing this you reduce the weight of the obstacle, little by little making it easier to move. In order to do this, you must deal with each issue individually, but you must first be able to identify its source.

To identify means to recognize somebody or something and to be able to say who or what he, she, or it is. When identifying someone there are different measures that can be taken. One can be identified through dental work, finger, hand, and footprints, voice recognition, hair samples, and also through their DNA. Another means of identification is using one's essential characteristics to define who they are. As you observe one's characteristics they reveal to you how they act, how they handle different situations, how they communicate, how they treat others, and what type of morals or scruples they have. So essentially it is because of their characteristics that you are able to recognize who they are, and the kind of nature they have. Each issue you've dealt with has its own separate identity or essential characteristics, that lets you know exactly what it is. If for example, you slip on something that causes you to fall, and break your leg and you notice that what you slipped on resembles a banana peel, tastes like a banana peel and smells like one, you have now recognized it by way of its essential characteristics, and can say without a doubt that the source of your broken leg is not the fall, but instead it is the banana peel. The fall is the issue that caused the broken leg, but it is not the source.

A source is the person, place, or thing through which something has come into being or existence, and everything and everyone that exists in this world has a source from which it or they have derived. Nothing that you can see, touch, taste, hear, or experience has come forth on its own, nor is it possible, and you should always be able to trace something, or someone to its origin or source. In order for you to heal emotionally and move forward with your life, it is imperative that you first properly identify the source of each painful event that have negatively impacted your life. Many times as human beings we will attempt to take a short cut to try and deal with issues we are faced with, but in doing so we find that we are never successful. This is because, when taking this route, we skip over steps that are a vital part of the process we must undergo, in order to reach our desired goal. When dealing with emotional issues, you'll find that the reason you are constantly chipping away at them, but never yielding positive results is because, you haven't gone back far enough to properly assess the situation.

Dealing with the source of a situation can be very time consuming, and difficult to say the least because it can require much research, which involves digging into various areas and turning over many stones before you can find out exactly where the situation began. This can be a very painful process that most people would rather skip over altogether, because often times when you trace a painful experience back to its root, you will find that in dealing with the source of one issue it will result in a spiraling path to something that you may have subconsciously blocked out. Usually it is something that was even more painful than what you're presently dealing with, and it is for this reason that many people resist digging into their past, because they're afraid of what they might find.

I call it the onion process. An onion is a round vegetable with thin dry skin and many layers inside that tastes and smells very strong. In attempting to peel back each layer of an onion because there are so many this process can be very tedious and time consuming. But before you can ever attempt to peel back the layers you must first go through the initial process, of cutting off the top skin and then cutting it in half or in quarters, but it is during this process that you must also endure a fine mist that escapes from the onion. As it escapes it gets into your eyes, causing them to burn and produce tears. And unless you put something on your face to protect your eyes this part of the process is totally unavoidable. Much like the onion some situations are very complex, and time consuming as well. In order to delve into the situation, and uncover all of the details needed to lead you to the source, there are many layers that must also be peeled back. Before you can attempt to peel back any of these layers you must first begin the initial process of dissecting the issue, but as you do this you begin to open up various areas of your life, revealing the truth of past events that you would much rather block out forever. As these memories begin to rise up before your eyes you experience a burning sensation in your heart, and this too can produce tears. When dealing with the painful experiences of past events, sometimes there is nothing you can do to prevent the tears, and this part of the process is also totally unavoidable.

Often times, because it is so hard for some people to face the truth of where their painful experiences originated, and because they have chosen to hold on to the past rather than seeking help, they deprive themselves of their healing. There are many people who have indeed chosen to continue to hold on to their issues, and it is almost as if they want to own what has happened to them. To own is to acknowledge full responsibility for something. The thing about owning something is that, whatever you own you must also bear the full weight of responsibility for it. It's no different than having a house full of children and being the sole provider, and because those children belong to you, all the weight of their cares falls totally on you and you alone. When you decide to own your issues, the full weight of everything that comes as a result of those issues also fall on you and you alone. You must maintain this thing all by yourself, and as long as you own it, it will continue to be a part of you and everything that you do.

We all have choices in life, and among those choices is the decision to either hold on to the past or let it go. If you choose to hold on to the past you are almost sure to suffer a lifetime of pain and agony, you will never be able to truly move forward, and your life will continue to hang in the balance. A balance is a state in which two opposing forces or factors are of equal strength or importance so that they cancel each other out and stability is maintained. So as you hold on to the past, because both your past and your future are opposing forces, and because each are of equal strength or importance, you not only cancel out your past but you also cancel out your future. The difference is, in a situation such as this there is no stability. When you hold on to the past you cancel out your future, because you cannot logically exist in between two places at the same time. So if for example you are in between two states, let's say Arizona and California, and if you are right at the border line of California but you continue to stand in that spot, this means that you will never enter California, but at the same time you are no longer in Arizona. So you are caught up somewhere in the middle of where you just left and where you want to be, but because you're not willing to let go of where you are and move forward you will go absolutely nowhere.

Usually, because of our own decisions something negative will happen to us, and much of the anger that is built up within us is because of this. People have a tendency to direct the anger they feel because of their own decisions toward someone else, but sometimes it's more of a sub-conscious act. There is an old adage that says, "to be human is to err, but to blame it on someone else is even more human", and in many cases people will blame someone else for their situation rather than face the fact of why they are where they are. This is because it is easier to blame others than it is to take responsibility for the part they have played. And though they might want to blame others for the condition of their life, the truth is that in many cases it is the decisions they've made that has caused their life to be in the state that it's in. So in seeking to identify the source of your issues the first place you need to look is within yourself. Once you have dealt with you, and have owned up to your own responsibility then you will be able to see clear enough to move on from where you are and deal with the source of your other issues, but it's possible that after searching within yourself you might find that there are no other sources.

You can't confront yourself without dealing with your pain, and you can't deal with your pain without eventually confronting yourself, and when it comes to healing, and deliverance it is usually harder to confront yourself than someone else. If you were to do an exercise where you stand before a mirror and confront yourself, you will probably have more questions than answers, and the answers that you do have will probably be the very ones you don't want to hear. Also as you stand there, you will have no one else to point your finger at, but if you do point it you'll find that the very finger you are pointing is pointing right at you.

Forgiving yourself is also a part of your healing and deliverance. One of the hardest things for people to do is to forgive themselves for the pain they have inflicted upon their self. What you need to understand is that it is equally as important for you to forgive yourself as it is for you to forgive others, because, until you forgive yourself it is impossible for you to move forward with your life. When you forgive yourself it's a win, win situation for you all of the way around, and you just might find that the un-forgiveness that you're holding against yourself is the biggest reason for most of the bondage you've been in. Sometimes as humans we can be our own worst enemy, and this is a very good example of how that happens. You have got to be able to admit you were wrong about some things and then love yourself enough to set you free from the prison of deception that you have built. Identifying the source of your pain isn't easy, and certainly isn't pleasant, but you must be willing to go through the entire process no matter what it takes, and no matter how long it takes.

In many cases when you are offended, just as you need to confront yourself, you also need to confront the individual that committed the offense. It's not always enough to just identify the source, but there are many times where it is absolutely necessary to confront the source of your offense before you can deal with the issue. While it sounds like a simple enough process that's not always the case, because it depends on who the offender is, and also whether or not they're still around for you to confront them. If you have ever been in this situation you understand what it's like to need to confront someone, but you can't because you have either lost contact, or they're deceased. This is one of the places where one can fall into the trap of holding grudges, and if you're not careful, it is also the moment that the door to a spiraling staircase of deep regret can be opened.

It is perfectly understandable to want to hold a grudge when someone deliberately hurts you, but the opposite of this is exactly what you need to do in order to receive your healing. As humans it is our first instinct to become angry and hold a grudge, but you need to understand that it is also very unhealthy for both your mind and your heart. When holding grudges if you're not careful you will begin to build a prison of offense around your mind, and at some point you can become so enraged that you will convince yourself that by holding on to unforgiveness you're somehow hurting the individual or individuals that hurt you, but the only purpose that it will serve is to have you bury the key which is needed to unlock the prison door, and set you free. Forgiveness is just as important for your own well-being as it is for the offender. For them it means the charges have been dropped, and they're no longer under the burden of guilt. But for you it means being set free from the weight of all of the mental stress that you are experiencing, as a result of everything that has built up in your heart.

Your freedom, healing and deliverance lies in your own hands, and just as it is with any source of information that you obtain, if you don't handle it properly it does you absolutely no good to have found it. So identify the source, deal with the issue and move on so you can enjoy the reward of a pain free life.

Medical Clause

As a point of information, and to protect myself from any possible lawsuit or criminal charges, I would like to make it known to my readers that I am not a psychologist, a counselor or a health professional of any kind. The next chapter of this book consists of data that was compiled from various medical websites, in an effort to share information with my readers that have already been made available to the public. I am in no way giving any medical advice or making any suggestions for anyone to do anything that is of a medical nature, nor am I attempting to diagnose anything whatsoever. If anyone believes, based on information cited in this or any other chapter in this book, that they could be suffering from an addiction, mental illness, or psychological and emotional trauma that is outlined in the next chapter, I strongly urge you to seek professional medical advice, so that you can receive an accurate medical diagnosis.

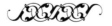

CHAPTER 7

Understanding the Source

OBTAINING THE WISDOM to identify the source of your pain is key, but in everything you receive if you don't have an understanding of what you're dealing with, the information you've obtained is primarily useless. When it comes to understanding the source it's important to know that there are two types of sources that you're dealing with. There is the main source and then there is the secondary source. The main source is the source or root cause of the issue that is causing the pain, and the secondary source is the issue itself. So you're dealing with the source of both the issue, and the pain, which is separate. It is important to also know that you can't just stop at gaining an understanding of the root cause of your particular issue and then ignore the issue itself, because before you can ever get to the root cause of an issue you must first gain an understanding of what type of issue you're dealing with. For example, you might be having crying spells, suicidal thoughts, bouts of sadness, feelings of emptiness and worthlessness, but these are not your issues they are symptoms, and some symptoms can be connected to more than one type of issue. So you have to look at the symptoms, figure out what is causing them, and then seek to know what caused you to develop the issue in the first place.

The following are dysfunctional behaviors or issues, along with a breakdown of the essential characteristics that will help you recognize whether or not this is something you might be struggling with and also the possible sources of the issues. Keep in mind that understanding what you're dealing with is the first step to winning the battle.

These behaviors or issues will be broken down under four different categories and are as follows:

Addictions

    Cutting and Self-harm

    Gambling Addiction/Problem Gambling

    Internet and Computer Addiction

    Pornography Addiction

    Sex Addiction

Substance Abuse Addictions

    Alcoholism/Problem Drinking

    Smoking Cessation

    Street Drugs and Prescription Drugs

Mental Health Illness

    Anxiety

    Bipolar Disorder

    Depression

    Eating Disorders (**Anorexia, Binge Eating, and Bulimia**)

    Obsessive-Compulsive Disorder

    Post-Traumatic Stress Disorder

    Schizoid Personality Disorder

    Schizophrenia

Emotional and Psychological Trauma

    Abandonment

    Caregiver Burnout Stress

Child Neglect and Abuse

Divorce/Breakup

Domestic Violence and Abuse

Elderly Abuse

Stress

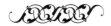

CHAPTER 8

Addictions

Cutting & Self-harm

Causes

CUTTING CAN BE a sign of someone under tremendous pressure and distress. They've found that this sort of dysfunctional behavior releases it, but it's also a behavior that some people outgrow.

Many times people have difficulty coping with their problems, and resort to cutting and harming themselves, in an effort to express feelings that they can't find a way to articulate, distract themselves from life as they know it to be and release themselves from their emotional pain. They may feel better for a while, however when the pain returns they feel the need to hurt them self again. One thing they need to keep in mind is that there are ways of feeling better without hurting their self.

Understanding cutting and self-harm

Harming yourself is a way of articulating and coping with deep sorrow and emotional pain. As unnatural as this may sound to those on the outside looking in, for some people hurting their self makes them feel better. In your mind you may feel like you have no choice, and that injuring yourself is the only way to cope with feelings of sadness, self-hatred, emptiness, guilt, and anger.

The problem with this is that though you might feel relief it is only temporary, and doesn't last long at all. It is equivalent to putting a Band-Aid on a cut that is in need of stitches. Though it stops the bleeding it is only temporary and instead of fixing the issue it only adds to the problem

If you're like the average person who resorts to self-injury, you will try to keep it a secret. This is probably because you feel ashamed or because you don't think anyone will understand. When you hide who you are and what you are feeling it becomes a heavy burden. The end result of this secret is that it causes you to feel guilty, and will begin to affect your relationships with your friends and family and also the way you feel about yourself. This mindset will only serve to make you feel even more alone, worthless, and imprisoned.

> **Why is it so difficult for children and teens to talk about cutting?**

Many times, children, by nature, want to try and handle it on their own.

They feel ashamed about it, and don't want to be controlled by their parents at this point.

They're trying to be more independent.

That's why open communication and acceptance is good.

> **Myths and facts about cutting and self-harm**

Self-harm tends to be difficult subjects to talk about, and many people harbor serious misconceptions about it, and the state of mind of the person that does it. One should not allow this to prevent them from getting the help they need.

Myth #1 People who cut and self-injure do it to get attention

Fact: The truth is that those who use self-harm usually do so in secret, and aren't trying to manipulate anyone, nor are they trying to draw attention to themselves. The shame and fear they feel makes it extremely difficult to come forward and ask for help.

Myth #2 People who self-injure are crazy and/or dangerous

Fact: The truth is that many who self-harm actually suffer from anxiety, depression or an earlier trauma. Self-injury happens to be how they cope, and accusing them of being crazy or dangerous is inaccurate and in addition it is not helpful.

Myth #3 People who self-injure want to die

Fact: In general, self-injurers usually have no desire to die. When they inflict harm on them self it is intended to help them cope with their pain, not kill them self. But it is a fact that those who self-injure do have a much higher risk of suicide, and this is why it is vital for them to get help.

Myth #4 Because the wounds aren't bad, it's not that serious

Fact: The deception is that because a person's wounds are not severe they aren't suffering much, but the severity of the wound does not determine how much that person is suffering, nor does it mean there is nothing to worry about.

➢ **Signs and symptoms of cutting and self-harm**

Signs that indicate your child may be in trouble

1. Have you noticed a sudden change in their friends, and the types of people they're hanging around? Have they withdrawn from their friends?
2. Have you noticed a difference in their school performance and grades? Have they withdrawn from activities they once loved?
3. Have their sleeping and eating patterns changed?
4. Do they have more angry outbursts or tearfulness?

Self-harm is anything you do to on purpose to injure yourself. Some of the more common ways of self-harm include:

- ❖ Cutting or clawing their skin
- ❖ Burning or scalding themselves

- ❖ Hitting their self or banging their head against something
- ❖ Punching things with their fists or slamming their body against walls or other hard objects
- ❖ Sticking pins, needles or other sharp objects into their skin
- ❖ Purposely preventing their wounds from healing
- ❖ Drinking poison or swallowing dangerous objects

Other less obvious measures of hurting oneself can include: reckless driving, drinking binges, taking too many drugs, and having unprotected sex.

➢ Warning signs of cutting or self-injuring

Clothing can always hide physical injuries, and a person can cover up their inner turmoil by remaining calm and at peace, and this can make self-harm hard to detect. But there are other things you can look for, and remember that you don't need hard evidence in order to reach out if you think someone is in trouble.

- ❖ Mysterious wounds or scars, from cuts, bruises, or burns, which are usually on the wrists, arms, thighs, or chest.
- ❖ Blood on their clothing, towels, or bedding and also blood-soaked tissues.
- ❖ A supply of sharp objects or cutting instruments, such as razors, knives, needles, broken pieces of glass, or bottle caps, in the person's belongings.
- ❖ Evidence of frequent accidents that they may try to explain away by claiming to be clumsy or having accidents.
- ❖ Covering themselves up, with long sleeves or long pants, even in hot weather.
- ❖ Claiming they need to be alone for long periods of time, especially in the bedroom or bathroom.
- ❖ Isolation and irritability.

➤ How cutting and self-harm helps

In your own words

- ❖ It expresses emotional pain or feelings that I feel on the inside, but am unable to put into words
- ❖ It's the only way I can think of for me to have control over my own body, since I can't control anything else in my life.
- ❖ I usually feel like I have a black hole in the pit of my stomach, feeling pain is better than feeling nothing at all
- ❖ I feel reassured and less anxious after I cut myself

If you didn't acknowledge the fact that self-harm is helpful you wouldn't be able to do it, therefore it is important to do so.

Some of the ways cutting and self-harming can help are as follows:

- ❖ Learning how to articulate feelings you can't put into words
- ❖ Learning how to release the pain and tension that's inside
- ❖ Helping you feel in control
- ❖ Diverting your attention from the overwhelming emotions or painful circumstances of life
- ❖ Relieving the guilt you feel and punishing yourself
- ❖ Making you feel alive, because the pain is better than feeling numb.

Once you gain an understanding of why you self-harm, then you will be able to learn different ways to stop self-harming, and also find resources to support you in winning this battle.

➤ If self-harm can help me, then why should I stop?

- ❖ While cutting and self-harm may give you temporary comfort, that comfort will come at a price, because if you do it long term it will produce more problems than it will ever solve.

- ❖ The relief you get from cutting and self-harm is short lived, and is also followed very quickly by feelings such as shame and guilt. In the meantime, it can hinder you from learning more effective approaches to recovery.

- ❖ Hiding cutting and self-harm from your friends and family members is both difficult and lonesome.

- ❖ Even though it's not your intentions to hurt yourself badly you can, because you can easily misjudge the depth of a cut, and wind up infecting the wound.

- ❖ You must learn other ways of dealing with your emotional stress, because if you don't it is guaranteed to put you at risk of having more difficult problems down the line. These problems include major depression, substance abuse, and suicide.

- ❖ Though cutting and self-harm may start off as something you do on a whim, or something that helps you maintain control over your circumstances, it can quickly become addictive, control your life, and become impossible to stop.

The bottom line is, self-harm and cutting will never be able to help you with the issues, that made you feel the need to hurt yourself in the first place.

➢ **Steps to recovery for cutting and self-harm**

Step 1 Confide in someone

➢ **Reaching out for help**

If you're in doubt about who or where to turn to for help, you may call the S.A.F.E. Alternatives hot line in the U.S. at **(800) 366-8288**. Upon calling you will be able to get both a referral and support, for cutting and self-harm. For helplines in other countries, see the resources and references below.

➢ **In a crisis**

If you're having suicidal thoughts, and you need immediate help, you may call the National Suicide Prevention Lifeline in the U.S. at **(800) 273-8255**. For a suicide helpline outside the U.S., visit Befrienders Worldwide, at **www.befrienders.org**.

If you have decided you're ready to get help for cutting or self-harm, **the first step is: to confide in someone else.** Sharing the very thing you've worked so hard to hide can be quite scary, however it can also be a great relief, to finally get to share your secret and confide in someone else concerning what you've been going through.

It can be very difficult trying to decide whom you can trust with such sensitive and personal information. Pick a person that you know will is not a gossiper, and who isn't going to try and control your recovery. Choose the one person in your life, who has accepted and supported you. That person could be one of the following: a teacher, best friend, your Pastor or other religious leader, a counselor or relative. It doesn't really have to be anyone that you're close to.

You may eventually desire to share your situation with those who are part of your inner circle, such as a close friend or family member. Many times it is easier to begin the process by confiding in an adult who you respect, like maybe one of your teachers, a church member, or your school counselor. These are people whom you can trust, but who at the same time is not so close to the situation, and therefore won't have a problem being objective.

➢ **Tips for talking about cutting and self-harm**

❖ **Focus on your feelings**

It's not necessary to share all of the fantastic details about your behavior, such as what exactly you do to hurt yourself, but it's more important to maintain your focus, on what lead you to hurt yourself. This will be key in helping the person you're sharing with, to gain a greater understanding of where you're coming from. This will also be helpful in letting them know exactly why you're telling them, for example, do you want their help or some advice, or is it that you simply want someone to unload the burden of your secret on?

❖ **Communicate in whatever way you feel most comfortable**

If you're nervous about talking to them in person, you might want to start the conversation off with an email or letter, and then do a face-to-face follow-up conversation. You don't have to feel like you're under any kind of pressure to share something you're not ready to talk about. In addition, there is no reason for you to think you must reveal your injuries, or answer any questions that you are not comfortable answering.

❖ **Give the person time to process what you tell them**

Though you might find it hard to open up and share your situation, it may be equally as difficult for the person you're confiding in to digest what you tell them, especially if it's someone you're very close to, such as family or a close friend.

There are times that you may not necessarily like how they react, but try and keep in mind that reactions such as shock, anger, and fear only present themselves because of their concern for you. The more information you can give them, the better they'll understand your addiction, and the better they will be able to support you.

It can be very stressful for you to talk about your addiction, and it will cause a lot of emotions to be stirred up. If you feel worse for a little while after you share your secret, but don't get discouraged about it. It's not altogether comfortable to face and alter long-standing habits, but once you begin the process and get past the initial stages, you will feel better.

Step 2 Figure out why you cut

➢ **Learning how to manage overwhelming stress and your emotions**

The first step toward recovering, is the vital process of understanding why you cut or self-harm. If you can learn what role self-injury plays in your particular case, you can then find other ways to get the job done, and at the same time minimize the desire to hurt yourself.

➢ **Identifying what triggers your self-harm**

It is important to keep in mind that; self-harm is generally a way of coping with emotional pain. What feelings most often make you want to cut or hurt yourself?

Is it sadness or is it anger? Could it be shame or could it be loneliness? What about guilt and emptiness?

The sooner you understand which of these feelings trigger your need to cut or self-harm, the sooner you will be able to begin developing healthier substitutes.

➢ Getting in touch with your feelings

If you're having trouble pinning down the feelings that trigger your desire to cut yourself, you might have to work on developing your mental alertness. This simply means, knowing what you feel and why you feel it. And that you have the ability to recognize and articulate what you feel from one moment to the next, and also to identify what connection there is between what you feel and your actions.

It will probably frighten you when you consider the idea of paying strict attention to what you're feeling, instead of using the usual self-harm numbing process. You may be concerned that you will become overwhelmed or get trapped in your distress. However, if you let go of your emotions you will find that they fade pretty quickly, being replaced by another one, as long as you don't beat yourself up, try and fight it, or judge yourself because of what you feel. Your feelings only linger when you persist in holding on to them.

Step 3 Finding new measures of coping

When you decide to stop cutting or harming yourself, you will need to have a substitute measure in place already, so that as you get a desire to hurt yourself you will be prepared to respond in a different manner.

If you cut so that you can express pain and intense emotions

- ❖ Begin painting, or drawing on a big sheet of paper, using red ink or paint
- ❖ Use a journal to express your feelings
- ❖ Write a poem or song to express what you feel
- ❖ As you experience these negative feelings write them down on a piece of paper, and then tear it up.
- ❖ Listen to music that you feel most expresses your emotions

If you cut so that you can calm and soothe yourself

- ❖ Soak in a bath or take a hot shower
- ❖ Spend time petting your dog or cat
- ❖ Wrap a warm blanket around yourself
- ❖ Get someone to give you a nice massage
- ❖ Listen to soothing music

If you cut because you feel unattached and dazed

- ❖ Call a friend and have a soothing conversation
- ❖ Jump in a cold shower
- ❖ Put a piece ice in the crook of your arm or leg
- ❖ Chew on something that has a very strong taste, such as: chili peppers, peppermint, or the peel of a grapefruit peel.
- ❖ Find a self-help website, and enter the chat room, or look at message board

If you cut because you need to release tension or vent anger

- ❖ Do rigorous exercises—run, dance, jump rope, or box
- ❖ Punch on something that won't hurt you or scream and vent
- ❖ Squeeze a stress ball or some Play-Doh
- ❖ Get a magazine or some paper and rip it up
- ❖ Make a lot of noise using pots, pans or an instrument

Other measures to use for the cutting sensation

- ❖ Use a red felt tip pen and put a mark on the spot where you would usually cut yourself
- ❖ Rub ice across the area on your skin where you would normally cut yourself

❖ Put rubber bands on your wrists, your arms, or your legs and when you get a sensation to cut, snap them instead

There is a great probability that as you work to overcome your addiction or habit you might also need the help and support of a trained professional. You might want to consider talking to a therapist. Therapists can assist you in developing new coping strategies and techniques to stop self-harming, while you work on getting to the root of why you cut or hurt yourself.

Remember, self-harm is an outward expression of inner pain that often takes root in early life. There is usually a connection between self-harm and childhood trauma. Many times self-harm will be your way of coping with feelings that are related to abuse from the past, flashbacks of the past abuse, negative feelings about how your body looks, or other traumatic experiences. Even if you're not aware of it there may still be a connection.

➢ **Finding the right therapy**

It might take some time to find the right therapist, but it's important that the one you choose has experience with treating both traumatic experiences and self-injury. Developing a quality relationship with your therapist is equally important, so trust your instincts, and if you don't feel safe, respected, or understood, find another one.

When choosing your therapist, there should always be a sense of trust and warmth between the two of you. This should be someone who can help treat you for self-harm without condoning it, and who is also willing to assist you in working toward stopping at your own pace. You should feel very comfortable talking with him or her, about your most personal issues.

Gambling addiction/problem gambling

Having a gambling addiction can and will put a strain on your relationships, cause problems with your employment, and also lead to financial ruin. In addition, it can cause you to do things you never imagined doing such as, stealing money both to gamble and to pay your bills. Just as with any other addiction, you can overcome it, but only after you recognize and acknowledge that you have a problem.

➤ Understanding gambling addiction and problem gambling

Gambling addiction, which is also known as compulsive gambling, is a type of impulse-control disorder. Compulsive gamblers have absolutely no control over their desire to gamble, even though they're aware that they are hurting themselves and those they love. Just as with other addictions gambling is all they think about, and the only thing they want to do, regardless of the problems it may cause. The thing about compulsive gamblers is that, it doesn't matter how they feel emotionally or what their financial circumstances are, they will still find a way to gamble. All of the odds can be stacked against them, and they can be in a situation where they can't afford to lose one more dollar, but the need to gamble will drive them to do it any way. With problem drinking you can have a problem and still be in control. Problem gambling is any gambling behavior that interferes your life.

Some signs of a gambling problem are: being preoccupied with it, spending more and more of your time and money to gamble, being convinced that you can win back what you've lost to the point of being obsessed with the pursuit of it, or being on the verge of losing things such as your family, your home or your job because of it.

Myths & Facts about Gambling Addiction and Problem Gambling

MYTH #1 If you're a gambler you have to do it everyday

Fact: This is not true. A problem gambler may gamble a few times a week or every day.

MYTH #2 If the gambler can afford to gamble they don't have a problem

Fact: As a Problem gambler, your problems are not limited to financial issues. If you spend an excessive amount of time gambling, it can cause you to lose a love relationship, business relationships and also valuable friendships.

MYTH #3 If you are a problem gambler, it is because you were driven to do so by your partners

Fact: People who have a gambling problem will blame it on someone else in an effort to rationalize their addiction, and to avoid taking responsibility for their own actions.

MYTH #4 If a problem gambler put their self in debt, you should help them pay it off

Fact: Wanting to help someone get out of a financial predicament is a noble thing to do, but instead of being a help you could potentially add to the problem by enabling them to continue with their addiction.

➢ **Alleviating negative and stressful feelings without gambling**

Dealing with unpleasant feelings such as tension, despair, loneliness, fear, and worry can either trigger compulsive gambling or make it worse. An occasional trip to the casino or the track can seem like a harmless, fun and exciting way to wind down, after a stressful day at work, an altercation with your spouse and even if you simply have a desire to socialize. But there are other things you can do to reach the same goal, such as exercising, hanging out with friends, finding a new hobby, or reading a nice book, without spending a lot of money.

If you are going to quit gambling it is essential to seek out other alternatives to dealing with the problems that you gamble to forget about. Even if you are successful in riding yourself of your gambling addiction, until you take the necessary measures to get rid of the problems that drove you to want to gamble, they will still exist. So it is important to put an offense mechanism in place to deal with the stressful situations that trigger your desire to gamble.

➢ **Signs and symptoms of problem gambling/gambling addiction**

A gambling addiction is often referred to as the "hidden illness" because you have no noticeable physical signs or symptoms such as those in drug or alcohol addiction. Problem gamblers are usually in deny the fact that they have a gambling addiction or they will make their problem seem a lot smaller than what it is. In addition, problem gamblers will go to great lengths to conceal their gambling, by getting money from family and friends, sneaking around, and lying about there whereabouts and activities.

➢ How can you know when you have a gambling problem?

You may have a gambling problem if you:

❖ Feel as if you need to keep your gambling a secret

You might lie and gamble in secret because you're concerned about whether or not others will understand your desire to gamble so much.

❖ Can't control your urge to gamble

You can't stop once you start gambling, or you feel obligated to gamble until all of your money is gone, continuing to raise your bets in an effort to win back what you've lost.

❖ Gamble even though you can't afford to

You are desperate to win back money you've lost, so you gamble until all of your money is gone and then start spending the money that is needed to pay your bills or by food and clothing for your children. You resort to borrowing, or stealing money or taking jewelry and other valuables to the pawnshop. You have convinced yourself that the only way you can win back the money you've lost is to continue gambling, but this only serves to put you further in debt.

❖ Your family and friends worry about you

If your family and friends are worried about you it is a good idea to listen, and then take a good look at how gambling has affected your life. Remember that asking for help does not mean you're weak. Don't be embarrassed to reach out to your adult children, even if you've gambled away what you had planned to leave as an inheritance for them and you feel they will be angry. It's never too late to make a positive change.

➢ Treatment for problem gambling

Because every gambler is unique they need a recovery program that is tailored to fit their specific needs. What works for one won't necessarily work for someone else. The first and biggest step in receiving treatment is acknowledging the fact that you have a gambling problem. Don't look at your situation as being hopeless, and don't try to do it alone. Many have dealt with this addiction, and have successfully kicked the habit. Although the process of quitting won't be easy, it is possible if you stick to your plan of treatment.

> **Group support for gambling addiction and problem gambling**

Gamblers Anonymous is a twelve-step program, much like Alcoholics Anonymous. One of the key parts of a twelve-step program is choosing a sponsor, which is a former gambler who has time and experience in remaining free from their gambling addiction, who's guidance and support can be priceless.

> **Therapy for problem gambling**

❖ **Cognitive-behavioral therapy**

Cognitive-behavioral therapy for gambling addiction concentrates on helping those addicted to change unhealthy gambling behaviors and thoughts, such as justifications and wrong beliefs. It also teaches them how to combat gambling urges, deal with unpleasant emotions rather than trying to escape their problems through gambling, and how to fix financial, work, and relationship problems that is a result of their addiction.

The goal of treatment is to retrain the gambler's brain by training them to think about gambling in a new way. A variation of cognitive behavioral therapy, called the Four Steps Program, has been used to treat compulsive gambling also. The goal of this type of therapy is to modify your beliefs and views about gambling in four separate steps; re-labeling, reattributing, refocusing, and revaluing. Seeing a therapist doesn't make you are weak nor does it mean you can't handle your problems. On the contrary, therapy is for those who are smart enough to realize they need help.

> **Maintaining recovery**

The act of quitting your gambling problem is relatively easy. The challenge is staying in recovery, and making a permanent commitment to stop gambling. Some of the things that can make maintaining your recovery possible is surrounding yourself with people that you're accountable to, avoiding environments that will tempt you to gamble, giving over control of your finances for a while, and finding other enjoyable activities to replace your gambling.

> **Modifying your routine and making healthier choices**

One way to handle your gambling problem is to recognize what triggers your gambling, work on ridding yourself of those elements and replace them with healthier options.

There are four elements that encourage gambling to continue and they are:

- **Decisions you make**

    In order for gambling to occur, one has to already have made a decision to gamble. If you find that you have an urge to gamble call someone, consider the consequences of your actions, and immediately find something else to do.

- **Having money available**

    If you don't have money, you can't gamble. Cancel your credit cards, let someone else manage your money, sign up for an automatic bill payment program with your bank, limit the amount of cash you carry on you at all times.

- **Making time for it**

    Gambling can only occur if you make the time for it. Make time for activities that have nothing to do with gambling, find time to relax, and plan recreational trips with your family.

- **Being at gambling establishments**

    Stay away from environments that tempt you to gamble. Tell the casino owners you have a problem and ask them to put restrictions on you while at their establishments. Block yourself from gambling sites on your computer.

The ability to maintain your recovery depends largely on the reasons why you gamble in the first place. Even after you've quit, if you gamble because of depression, loneliness, or boredom unless you address these issues prior to quitting they will remain, and hinder your recovery.

➤ Dealing with the urge to gamble

Resisting cravings will become easier for you, as you make healthier options and develop a good support system.

Using the following strategies can help you

- **Seek support**

    Reach out to a trusted family member, or friend or find a Gamblers Anonymous support group.

- **Find something else to do**

    Preoccupy your mind by doing things like cleaning your house, exercising, or watching a movie.

- **Postpone your trip to the casino**

    Prolong your trip for as long as you can, if you can wait long enough your urge to gamble may become weaker, allowing you to resist going altogether.

- **Give yourself a reality check**

    Think about what could happen if you give in to the desire to gamble. Consider how you will feel after losing all of your money, how disappointed your family will be and the damage it could do to your relationship with them.

- **Avoid being alone**

    If socializing or being around other people is your reason for gambling, look for other ways to build a social network, such as volunteering, making new friends or connecting with old ones.

Overcoming a gambling addiction is not an easy process, so if you find that you can't resist this craving, don't be so hard on yourself and don't use it as an excuse to give up.

Even though you might slip up sometimes it is important that you learn from your mistakes and keep moving forward with your recovery.

Preventing suicide in problem gamblers

The risk of suicide can be quite high for gamblers when they begin to feel hopeless. If they are talking about suicide it is important that you take it very seriously. If you or someone you know is suicidal, call the National Suicide Prevention Lifeline at **1-800-273-8255**. For a suicide helpline outside the U.S., visit Befrienders Worldwide.

➢ **Tools for loved ones of problem gamblers**

❖ **Start by helping yourself**

It is important to understand that you have a right to protect yourself emotionally and financially. Without losing yourself in the process, find someone who can help you make the right choices for yourself, while encouraging your loved one to get help.

❖ **Don't go it alone**

When coping with a loved one's gambling problem it can become so overwhelming, that you may feel it's easier to just excuse their problem one last time. Feeling as if you're the only one that is dealing with such a problem, can cause you to feel ashamed, but in reaching out for help you are likely find, that there are other families struggling with it too. Keep in mind, that therapy is always an option for you and can be very helpful.

❖ **Set boundaries when it comes to managing money**

If a loved one is serious about getting help, suggest taking over the finances for a while to keep them accountable and help prevent them from relapsing. In taking on the responsibility of ensuring that your finances and credit is safe, understand that this does not mean you have to micromanage your loved one's gambling problem.

❖ **How to respond to requests for money**

Just as with any other addiction, problem gamblers can be very good at getting money to satisfy their urge to gamble, either directly or indirectly. They may use such techniques as pleading, manipulation, threats and even the blame game to get it. It will take you some time and practice to learn how to deal with these requests, ensuring that you are not enabling your loved one and keeping your own dignity intact in the process.

[Internet or Computer Addiction]

Using the Internet has its place and can be very productive, but when it becomes compulsive it can interfere with daily life, work, and relationships. If you find that you feel more comfortable with your face book friends than your real ones, or you find it difficult to stop playing games, gambling or consistently checking your smartphone, tablet, or other mobile device, even though you know it will have very negative consequences in relationships, at school or on your job, you're spending too much time on the Internet.

➢ **What is Internet or computer addiction?**

Internet Addiction, which is also known as computer addiction, online addiction, or Internet addiction disorder (IAD), covers a number of impulse-control problems, which includes:

❖ **Cybersex Addiction**

This consists of obsessive use of pornography found on the Internet, chat rooms for adults only, or adult fantasy role-play sites that has a very negative impact on real-life intimate relationships.

❖ **Cyber-Relationship Addiction**

This is an addiction to social networking, chat rooms, texting, and messaging, to the point where simulated online friends, have become more important to someone than real-life relationships with their loved ones and friends.

- ❖ **Net Compulsions**

    This addiction results in compulsive online gaming, on-line gambling, stock trading or compulsive on-line auction sites like eBay, and usually causes huge financial and job-related issues.

- ❖ **Information Overload**

    This is an addiction that causes compulsive web surfing or database searching. This can lead to a lesser work output, and also lesser social communication with loved ones and friends.

- ❖ **Computer Addiction**

    This addiction results in a compulsive need to play off-line computer games, like Solitaire, or compulsive computer programming.

Of these addictions, the most common ones are cybersex, on-line gambling and cyber-relationship addiction.

> **Healthy Internet use vs. unhealthy Internet use**

The Internet is very valuable, and provides a consistent, source of information and entertainment that changes continuously. Internet information can be retrieved from almost every smartphone, tablets and laptops, desktop computers and email, blogs and social networks, and, instant messaging and message boards. These modes of communication allow for both public, and anonymous communication about any topic. But the question is, how much is too much Internet usage?

Internet usage for each person is different. For example, you might need to use the Internet significantly for your job, or you may rely greatly on social networking sites in order to stay in touch with family and friends who are far away. It is not until your time spent on the Internet begins to absorb too much of your time, causing you to neglect your relationships, work, school, and everything else that's important in your life, that it becomes a problem for you. If you continue to display this type of behavior despite the negative consequences you face in life, then it's time to find a new equilibrium.

> **Causes of Internet or Computer Addiction**

People become addicted to the Internet to relieve unpleasant and overwhelming feelings

Many people resort to Internet addiction in order to deal with unpleasant feelings such as tension, loneliness, hopelessness, and anxiety. When they have a bad day, and begin searching for a way to flee from their problems, or to quickly ease their tension, the Internet can be an easily reachable outlet. Losing yourself online can temporarily make feelings like loneliness, stress, agitation, despair, and boredom disappear into thin air, and even though the Internet has the ability to provide much comfort, you must keep in mind that there are much healthier ways to manage negative feeling and keep them in check. Some of them include exercise, meditation, and simple relaxation techniques.

The quickest resolution to overcoming Internet and computer addiction is to discover other ways to deal with these negative feelings. Though your Internet usage may appear to be normal again, unless you take the time to deal with your stressful issues and the things that irritate you on a daily basis, those negative feelings will continue to remain, having the ability to once again prompt you to rekindle an unhealthy relationship with the Internet and your computer.

> **Risk factors for Internet addiction and computer addiction**

You are at greater risk of Internet addiction if:

- **You suffer from anxiety**

    Use of the Internet helps to distract you from your fears and concerns. An anxiety disorder like obsessive-compulsive disorder may also be a contributing factor to excessive email checking and compulsive Internet use.

- **You are depressed**

    Though many use the Internet to flee from illnesses such as depression, spending too much time on-line can make things worse. Internet addiction can have a reverse affect and actually wind up further contributing to stress, isolation and loneliness.

- ❖ **You have other addictions**

    Many Internet addicts suffer from other addictions, such as drugs, alcohol, gambling, and sex.

- ❖ **You lack social support**

    On-line gaming, social Networking and instant messaging is a safe way for Internet addicts to establish new relationships and also become more confident in their ability to relate to others.

- ❖ **You're an unhappy teenager**

    If you have a problem fitting in, the Internet can be a place of comfort for you, making it easier to communicate with on-line friends rather than real-life friends.

- ❖ **You are less mobile or socially active than you once were**

    Your ability to drive or leave the house has been severely limited, due to a disability or the lack of a baby sitter.

- ❖ **You are stressed**

    If not careful the Internet can be counterproductive, because while you may use it to relieve stress, the longer you stay on it the higher your stress levels can be.

- ➢ **Signs and symptoms of Internet addiction or computer addiction**

Signs and symptoms of Internet addiction will vary from person to person. There is nothing in particular that would indicate a person might be addicted to the Internet. But here are some general warning signs that you can look for, to let you know that your Internet use may have become a problem:

- ❖ **Losing track of time while online**

    You are frequently on the Internet longer than you intended. A few minutes of intended use on the Internet turns in to a few hours. When your Internet time is interrupted you get irritated.

❖ **You're having trouble finishing jobs at work or home**

You find that your laundry begins to pile up, and you have very little food in the house because you've been too busy using the Internet. You end up working late because of your inability to complete your tasks on time, and you begin to use not finishing your tasks as an excuse to stay longer at work, so that you can use the Internet uninterrupted.

❖ **Isolating yourself from family and friends**

Your social life is suffering because you spend too much time online. Your family and friends are being neglected. You feel like no one in your life understands you like your Internet friends.

❖ **You're feeling guilty or defensive about your Internet use**

You are irritated because your spouse asks you to get off the computer or smartphone and spend time with them. You've begun hiding your Internet use, and lying to your boss and family about how much time you spend on the computer or mobile devices, as well as what you do while you're online.

❖ **You are full of joy while involved in Internet activities**

You've begun using the Internet as an outlet whenever you feel stressed, or sad and for sexual pleasure. You have been unsuccessful in every attempt to limit your Internet usage.

➢ **Physical symptoms**

Internet or computer addiction can cause physical distress such as:

❖ Carpal Tunnel Syndrome, consisting of pain and numbness in hands the and wrists

❖ Dry eyes or strained vision

❖ Back, and neck aches along with severe headaches

❖ Unable to sleep

❖ Noticeable weight gain or weight loss

➤ Internet addiction: Cybersex and pornography

Pornography and cybersex addictions are really types of sexual addiction. But because it is on the Internet it makes it easier to access, while allowing you to remain relatively anonymous. One can easily spend hours on the Internet, engaging in fantasies that are impossible in real life, in the privacy of their own home.

Your real-life relationships, your career, and your emotional health can all be negatively impacted, because of your Compulsion to spend so much time on the Internet, viewing pornography and engaging in other cybersex activities.

➤ The difference between healthy and unhealthy sexuality

For most adults, healthy sexuality is usually a mixture of sexual practices. Sex with a partner, or as a part of exploring or discovering new relationships is usually an enjoyable act of choice. However, when it comes to sexual addicts, sexual conduct can usually be described by words such as obsessed, compulsive, and concealed. Healthy sex is usually a practice between two people in a relationship, but sexual addicts use sex as a way of coping, dealing with boredom, worry, and other dominant feelings or they use it as a means to make them feel significant, desired, or strong.

➤ Internet addiction: Online gambling

While the art of gambling has been a widely recognized problem for years, the accessibility of Internet gambling has made it much more accessible. It has also made it much more difficult for recovering addicts to prevent having a relapse. Online or virtual casinos are open 24 hours, and are accessible for anyone with Internet access. This venue to gambling has made it much easier for those who don't live close to a casino, and even those who are too young to otherwise gain access to gamble on-line.

➤ Other Internet compulsions

Net compulsions such as stock trading, or online auction shopping venues can be just as damaging as online gambling. This makes it easy for those that are eBay addicts, to wake up at strange hours and get online for the last remaining minutes of an auction. It enables them to make purchases that they don't need, and can't afford, just so they can experience the thrill of placing what could be the winning bid.

Compulsive online gamers have the ability to isolate themselves for many hours at a time, neglecting different areas of their lives while taking part in virtual reality or online fantasy games.

➢ Internet addiction: Cyber-relationships

When it is used responsibly, the Internet can be a really great place to have social interaction, meet new people, and possibly even start intimate relationships. However, much of the time, online relationships can be a lot more intense than real-life relationships. People remove all boundaries, allowing their fantasies to have free reign and for some the very idea of spending time with their online love can far exceed all sensible expectations. Very few real-life relationships have the ability to compete with these wild, fantasy relationships, therefore the Internet addict will almost always prefer to spend more and more time on-line with their fantasy friends.

Some other problems that you can run in to is that, around 50% of those who are online will lie about their age, weight, job, marital status, or their gender. When you finally meet your on-line friend, and find that they're not what or who they said they are, this can cause great emotional disappointment and distress.

➢ Self-help tips for ending an Internet addiction

There are many steps you can take to manage your Internet use, and get it under control. While you can start many of these steps on your own, it would be wise to get outside support, because it can very easy to fall back into your old patterns of usage, and this is especially so if you have to use the Internet a lot for work or other needful activities.

Try to identify the main problems that may support your Internet addiction

Are you struggling with depression, stress, or tension? Is Internet addiction a way to self-soothe your bad moods? Have you struggled with alcohol or drugs in the past? Do you feel a need to use Internet to numb yourself in the same way that you used alcohol when you used to drink? Try to identify if you need to get treatment in these areas or if you need to return to group therapy.

- ❖ **Build your coping skills**

    Internet may be your way of coping with stress or anger, or you might be very shy and have a difficult time relating to other people. If you can build coping skills it may help you deal with your stressful moments throughout the day without having to rely on Internet use to do it.

- ❖ **Strengthen your network of support**

    The more real-life relationships you have, the less Internet interaction you will need. Dedicate yourself to setting aside quality time each week for your friends and family. If you are shy, get connected with groups that you have things in common with, such as sports, education, or reading. You will be able to develop relationships naturally, as you interact with others.

➢ **Revising your Internet & computer use step by step:**

So that you can monitor your problem areas, keep a daily journal, of how often you are on the Internet for leisure or non-essential activities. Monitor whether or not there are specific times of the day, that you use the Internet more than others. What are the things that trigger you during the day, to stay ne the Internet for hours at a time, when you've only planned to be on for a few minutes?

- ❖ Set a schedule to use the Internet. For example, try setting a timer, scheduling certain times of the day, or making a vow to turn off your computer, tablet, or smartphone at a certain time each day.

- ❖ Instead of getting on the Internet, replace that time with healthy activities. Since it's the times when you're bored, and lonely, that it's hardest to resist the urge of getting on the Internet, make a plan of other ways to fill the time.

➢ **Tips for dealing with Internet addiction:**

- ❖ Ask yourself what you're missing out on, by spending so much time on the Internet. Write down these activities and slowly return to them, while decreasing your Internet time.

- ❖ Set reasonable times for the Internet and stick to them. Take breaks often, and find other activities to get involved in.

- ❖ Change your routine in order to break your normal patterns of usage. For example, if you're on-line in the evenings, start limiting your use to mornings only.

- ❖ Hang out with people you know, who are rarely on the Internet. Take the time to value the life without the Internet.

- ❖ Stay connected to the real world. Purchase a regular newspaper, read paperback book, and listen to CD's from a CD player. Go to Theatre's to watch plays and movies and visit museums.

- ❖ Use the Internet as it is meant to be used; as a tool. Remember that the Internet is only a means to an end. Plan your strategy for getting on the Internet, whether you're looking for information or entertainment.

➢ **Treatment, counseling, and support**

- ❖ **Cognitive-behavioral therapy** delivers step-by-step measures to put an end to compulsive Internet behaviors, and change your views concerning Internet, smartphone, and computer use. In addition, therapy can help you find healthier ways of dealing with negative emotions, such as tension, anxiety, or depression.

If your Internet use is directly affecting your spouse, marriage counseling can be very helpful, while trying to work through these challenging issues. It can also help you relink with your spouse, if the Internet has been taking the place of most of your social needs.

➢ **Group support for Internet addiction**

Internet addiction is relatively new therefore, it can be hard to find a real-life support group that is committed to the issue. But there may be groups where you can work on social and coping skills, such as for anxiety or depression. SAA or Sex Addicts Anonymous may be another place to try if you are experiencing problems with cybersex.

Ironically, there are some Internet addiction support groups on the Internet. But these sites should be used with caution. They may be helpful in positioning you and pointing you in the right direction, but you still need real-life people in order to truly benefit from group support.

Pornography Addiction

A porn addiction is often quite difficult to diagnose. Although many people can use porn simply for the purpose of spicing up their relationships, others may become obsessive or even compulsive porn users. Those who fall in the last category probably suffers from a porn addiction. Pornography addiction may cause you to decrease the amount of time spent socializing, while causing you to be you sexually unresponsive. If your partner has become increasingly insistent or unusually rough during intercourse, this could indicate they're struggling with a porn addiction.

> **Causes of Porn Addiction**

There are many different factors that can cause a sex addiction. Some of the causes can include depression and anxiety, but sex addiction can also stem from by sexual abuse. There are many people that are addicted to sex, and during sexual intercourse or other sex-related activities they experience brain stimulation, and over a period of time, one can become addicted to these feelings.

It is quite difficult to have a healthy relationship with sex addict, and especially if your partner is addicted to porn. A porn addiction will interfere with one's ability to have a normal, and healthy relationship. If your partner is impulsively watching porn, even as you're attempting to be intimate with him or her then it has their attention and not you. In other words, their relationship with porn is more important to them, than their relationship with you. It's not really any different than having an outside affair.

It's no secret that some couples use porn together, in order to light a fire under a relationship that's suffering or to add some variety and pleasure. If you have a mutual agreement and are viewing it together, that's totally different from having

Healing the Hurts of Yesterday

an addiction to porn, unless, of course, both of you have become obsessed with it and your relationship has begun to suffer as a result.

It's possible that your partner is addicted to pornography, and though you couldn't quite put your finger on it, you've sensed that something is wrong. The one thing you know for sure is that your relationship is no longer fulfilling, at least not for you and if it is going to continue something will have to change.

➢ Signs of Pornography Addiction

There are several signs that can serve as an indicator, that you may have a sex addiction. Some symptoms are emotional, but many are physical as well.

The following are 6 signs that you have a porn addiction. If you have noticed some of these signs, but haven't noticed others don't ignore it.

- ❖ **You have become reserved** If you were once socially active, but have begun making excuses to avoid group activities, is spending an unusual amount of time online, or is spending more and more time alone, it could be because you are obsessed with porn.

- ❖ **You are spending an excessive amount of time online**

    Those who have an addiction to sex usually use the Internet to gratify their desire for more. This supply is basically endless and much of it is free. If you have been secretive, and try to hide what you've been watching or you're suddenly using the Internet regularly, either late at night or early in the morning while your partner is sleeping, this should send up even more red flags.

- ❖ **You seem mentally unattached from your relationship**

    Often this is more noticeable during sex, where you're together physically, but you are seemly somewhere else mentally and don't seem to care, that your partner is feeling less fulfilled.

- ❖ **you criticize your partner's body or overall appearance**

    Most porn stars have exceptional bodies (which have been surgically enhanced), and are often very young and firm. The more time you spend looking at them, the more unfavorably you're going to look at your partner, comparing them to the actors and models you've been looking at for hours. You have almost no desire for sex, and if you do have sex, your partner must initiate it. In addition, you don't seem to be into it while having sex. You're not giving much in return, seem to be going through the motions, and your level of arousal is very low in comparison to what it used to be like.

❖ **Your partner's sexual tastes have changed**

In the beginning of your relationship you were very well matched sexually, and now it's like you're someone totally different. You want to try things that are new and unusual, with which your partner isn't comfortable. You even resort to talking and acting differently while you're having sex. You are rougher, more insistent, and essentially treating them like an object instead of someone you love.

❖ **Your partner is evasive, defensive, lying or secretive**

Because of your addiction to porn your relationship is suffering, you're not being honest with them and shut them out. If they attempt to talk about it, you either become vague or gets defensive. You begin hiding pornography from your partner, keeping a private email address, and also spending money on pornography, while lying about it.

➢ **Other signs of an addiction to porn may include:**

  ❖ Mood changes and an increased detachment
  ❖ A decrease in time spent on other activities
  ❖ Less time spent with others
  ❖ Increase in amount of time spent using pornography
  ❖ Less amount of time spent taking care of personal responsibilities
  ❖ An increase in risk of unprotected sexual encounters
  ❖ Partaking in use of drugs or alcohol to heighten sexual experiences

- **4 progressive steps that a porn addict generally goes through are:**
  - **Addiction** - Compulsively viewing pornography.
  - **Escalation** – Over a period of time, the addict will require more extreme and abnormal material in order to get the same effect and satisfy their sexual urges.
  - **Desensitization** - The addict will lose their ability to discern what is socially acceptable, and material that is considered to be illegal, unthinkable, immoral, or disgusting to most people will seem normal to them.
  - **Acting out sexually** – They will develop an increased tendency to act out the sexual performances that they view in pornography, and take part in other activities such as uncontrollable promiscuity, exhibitionism, orgies, voyeurism, increased visits massage parlors, sex with minors, rape and even causing pain on themselves or their partner during sex.
  - **Consequences of porn addiction include:**
  - Your Intimate relationships are greatly damaged
  - Increased sense of self shame and guilt
  - Interference with work, school and job
  - Financial problems
  - Legal troubles
  - Greater risk of divorce
  - Increased risk of sexually transmitted diseases
- **Pornography Addiction Treatment**

Addiction changes the neurotransmitters that are naturally produced in the brain, regulating communication between the cells, muscles, and organs, and also distorts brain functioning. People addicted to pornography, should be treated by medical professionals that are knowledgeable of addictive behavior.

The two sides of addiction are: the physical and psychological side. The emotional trait of this addiction has to be looked at closely and then treated, if one is to return to a healthy sexual behavior. It is just as crucial to pay attention to the individual, group and family therapy, as it is for the physical addiction.

Withdrawal symptoms could accompany the interruption of the behavior that is linked with porn addiction. For a person that is addicted there are a number of things they need to learn such as the following:

- The nature of addiction
- The people, places, and things that can trigger a return to addictive behavior
- Stress reduction techniques
- Self-estimated behavior and a host of other addiction related issues that can help a person manage abstinence.

Many times, a person that is suffering from this addiction will also suffer from a mental disorders such as:

- Anxiety
- Depression
- Antisocial behavior
- Obsessive-compulsive disorder
- Drug or alcohol addiction

Under these circumstances, it is important to make a proper diagnosis so that all addictions and mental disorders can be treated. The treatment for pornography addiction may fall under the broader scope of treatment used for sexual addiction. Whether a person receives inpatient or outpatient treatment will be determined by their mental and physical health. After a full evaluation and a proper diagnosis, if it is found that they suffer from a mental health disorder, and/or a drug or alcohol addiction, they will most likely receive an anti-depressant. Porn addiction treatment arms the addict with the knowledge needed to make healthy choices for their life.

Unlike drugs and alcohol addictions, most insurance companies won't cover treatment for pornography addiction, but there are several organizations that can guide porn addicts through the recovery process.

Some facilities including SRI or Sexual Recovery Institute offer online services for sexual addiction treatment. Nearly all of the 12 step sexual addiction programs offer on line support group meetings, and weekly sexual recovery chats. Two of the 12 step organizations that are known to address this type of addiction are Sex Addicts Anonymous and Sex and Love Addicts Anonymous.

Sexual Addiction

> **What is a sexual addiction?**

Sexual addiction is best described as a progressive intimacy disorder, characterized by compulsive sexual thoughts and acts. Like all addictions, its negative impact on the addict and on family members increases as the disorder progresses. Over time, the addict usually has to intensify the addictive behavior in order to achieve the same results.

Sex addicts don't automatically become sex offenders, and all sex offenders are not sex addicts. Only about 55 percent of those convicted of sexual assault can be considered as sex addicts, but 71 percent of those who molest children are sex addicts. Many sex addicts have such severe problems that imprisonment is the only way to make sure that those in our society are safe from them. More than 30 million people are thought to suffer from a sexual addiction in the United States alone, and our society has accepted the fact that sex offenders don't rape to receive sexual gratification, but instead they do it out of a troubled need to have power, control, revenge, or some warped expression of anger.

Just like eating, sex is both natural and necessary for human survival. There are people who are celibate for many reasons. Some are, not by any choice of their own, and others choose to be celibate for cultural or religious reasons, but whatever the reason, healthy humans have a strong desire for sex. As a matter of fact, a lack of interest or a low interest in sex can indicate either a medical problem or a psychiatric illness.

➢ Types of Sexual addictions

Paraphilic & NonParaphilic

Paraphilias are disorders where the addict becomes sexually aroused, by objects or actions that are considered unusual, and are not easily accessible to the sex addict. Examples of paraphilias include fetishism (arousal by objects or specific body parts), voyeurism (arousal by watching sexual behaviors), exhibitionism (arousal by having others view his or her sexual behaviors) and pedophilia (arousal by sexual contact with children). Some people with sex addictions never advance beyond the more easily accessible addictive acts such as, having one night stands, multiple affairs, contact with prostitutes, chat rooms, personal ads, obsessive masturbation, pornography, or phone or computer sex. But for others, addiction may include unlawful activities such as making obscene phone calls, or rape.

Non-paraphilic addictions, are classified by the Diagnostic, and Statistical Manual of Mental Disorders (*DSM*) as sexual disorder, not otherwise specified.

➢ Causes of sexual addiction

There is no one factor that is thought to cause sexual addiction, however some think there are biological, psychological, and social factors that add to the growth of these illnesses. One possible cause is intoxication that is thought to be the result of alterations in chemicals and certain regions in the brain that are caused by the compulsion.

Psychological risk factors for sexual addiction include depression, anxiety and obsessive-compulsive inclinations. It is also thought that learning disability increases the risk of one acquiring a sex addiction. Others who suffer with this disorder have personality traits like insecurities, impulsivity, compulsive behavior, problems maintaining stable relationships and intimacy, the inability to tolerate irritation, as well as problems coping with their emotions. In addition, those who have been sexually abused are at a higher risk of forming a sexual addiction.

➢ Signs and symptoms

Although the *DSM* have not come up with any specific investigative criteria for non-paraphilic sex addictions, some have suggested using signs and symptoms that are akin to other addictions, for paraphilic sex addictions and non-paraphilic sex addictions. Sex addicts in particular, have been labeled as someone suffering from a negative type of sexual behavior that points to major issues or distress that may include:

- ❖ A need for a greater intensity of behavior to attain the desired outcome.
- ❖ Withdrawing physically or psychologically because of the inability to be involved in the addictive behavior.
- ❖ The addict making plans for, or engaging in these sexual behaviors longer than they originally planned.
- ❖ Not being able to cut back or cease from their sexual behavior.
- ❖ Not engaging in important group, work, or school activities because of their sexual behavior.
- ❖ Continuing to engage in their sexual activities regardless of the physical or psychological consequences.

➢ Emotional Symptoms of Sex Addiction

If you suffer from a sex addiction, you probably won't have healthy boundaries. You will become very easily involved with people sexually or emotionally even if you don't really know them.

Because most sex addicts have a fear of being abandoned, you will most likely stay in relationships that aren't healthy, or you will probably jump from one relationship to another. When you're alone, you will tend to feel empty or lacking.

➢ Physical Symptoms of Sex Addiction

Although a sex addiction can create many physical side effects, there are few physical symptoms. But you might notice that you feel powerless due to an obsession with sexual or emotional desires.

➢ Diagnosing Sexual Addiction

Just as true as it is with pretty much any other mental-health diagnosis, there is no one test that conclusively indicates, that someone has a sexual addiction. Because of this, health-care physicians detect these disorders by collecting complete medical, family, and mental-health information to separate sexual addiction from medical and other mental-health disorders. A Physical examination will be performed by, a psychologist, psychiatrist, social worker, certified counselor, or psychiatric nurse. It may also be requested of the person's primary physician to do the exam. The exam will consist will of tests used to evaluate an individual's general health, to determine whether or not they have a medical illness that has mental-health indicators.When assessing a person who is thought to have a sexual addiction, mental-health professionals are checking to see if the individual is suffering not only from sexual obsession or compulsion, but also from mental illnesses such as depression or manic depression symptoms. Due to the fact that some of the symptoms of sex addiction can also show up in other mental illnesses, the mental-health screening is given to find out if the individual is suffering from mental-health disorders such as:

Panic disorder, generalized anxiety disorder, posttraumatic stress disorder (PTSD), the cyclical mood swings of bipolar disorder, attention deficit hyperactivity disorder (ADHD). Any disorder that is associated with hypersexual behavior, like developmental disorders, borderline personality disorder, dependent personality disorder, antisocial personality disorder, or multiple personality disorder (MPD).

In order to accurately determine if a person has a sexual addiction, health-care physicians must work to differentiate sexual addictions from medical conditions that just might include hypersexual warning signs. Some of the examples include seizures, tumors, dementia, and Huntington's disease, which could involve injuries to certain regions of the brain such as the frontal or temporal lobes and therefore influence behavior.

➢ Treatment for sexual addiction

If you have a sexual addiction you may benefit from the support and structure of recovery groups like Sex Addicts Anonymous and Sexaholics Anonymous. The use of cognitive behavioral therapy exists to assist individuals with sex addiction, in learning what triggers their sexually destructive behavior, doing a reevaluation of the distorted thoughts that contribute to their damaging behaviors, and that will eventually control those behaviors. Sexual addictions can become so severe that they may require going to an inpatient treatment center or an intensive outpatient program.

Serotoninergic (SSRI) are medications that are generally used to treat depressive and anxiety disorders, as well as mood stabilizers that are used to treat bipolar disorder, have been proven to reduce the compulsive longings linked with sexual addictions for some addicts.

Some of the SSRI's include:

Fluoxetine a generic name for **Prozac**

Paroxetine a generic name for **Paxil,**

Sertraline a generic name for **Zoloft,**

Citalopram a generic name for **Celexa,**

Fluvoxamine a generic name for **Luvox,**

Escitalopram a generic name for **Lexapro**

SSRIs are usually tolerated pretty well, and have mild side effects. Some of the usual side effects include: nausea, diarrhea, agitation, insomnia, and headache. But hey usually go away sometime during the first month of taking SSRI. Some of the sexual side effects are, decreased sexual desire aka decreased libido, delayed orgasm, or an inability to have an orgasm. Some patients have been known to experience tremors when taking SSRIs.

Mood stabilizers like carbamazepine (Tegretol), divalproex sodium (Depakote), and lamotrigine (Lamictal) are sometimes used to treat individuals with OCD, and particularly those who also suffer from bipolar disorder. These medicines could also be helpful in reducing the compulsive behaviors that are suffered by some sex addicts.

Naltrexone is a medication that is generally used to reduce the effects of narcotic medications, but could be useful for reducing the sexual compulsions, sex drive, or arousal of some sex offenders. This medicine could be particularly valuable for people who have a sexual addiction and have sought out celibacy to refrain from their sexual compulsions.

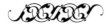

CHAPTER 9

Substance Abuse Addiction

Alcohol Abuse/Alcoholism

Because alcohol abuse and alcoholism has the ability to sneak up on you, it is very important to know all of the warning signs, and also to be wise enough to take the necessary steps to pull back once you recognize them.

> **Understanding Alcohol Abuse/Alcoholism**

Main source:

- ❖ Genetics, how one was raised, their social environment, and their emotional health are all interrelated factors that cause alcoholism and alcohol abuse.
- ❖ It is said that certain racial groups such as American Indians, and Native Alaskans are more at risk of developing an alcohol addiction.
- ❖ People whose family has a history of alcoholism and those who associate with heavy drinkers are more at risk.
- ❖ Those who suffer from various mental health conditions such as bipolar, depression, and anxiety are also more susceptible to become addicted to alcohol because it can be used to self-medicate.

➢ Hints of problematic drinking

You could potentially have a drinking problem if you:

- ❖ Feel guilty or ashamed about how much you drink
- ❖ Lie about or hide your drinking habits
- ❖ Have loved ones who are concerned about the fact that you drink
- ❖ Have to drink to relax or feel better
- ❖ Black out and forget things you've done while drinking
- ❖ Often find yourself drinking more than you set out to consume

Drinking is very common in many nationalities and effect everyone differently, therefore it's not always easy to identify the line that divides social and problem drinking. It just depends upon how it affects you as an individual. If your alcohol consumption impacts your life in a negative fashion, it is safe to say you have a drinking problem.

➢ Signs and Symptoms of Alcohol Abuse

The main distinction between alcoholism and alcohol abuse is known as alcohol dependence. **Alcohol dependence** is a substance-related disorder in which an individual is addicted to alcohol either physically or mentally, and continues to use alcohol despite significant areas of dysfunction, evidence of physical dependence, and/or related hardship. Alcoholics are dependent on alcohol and alcohol abusers, although they may have the ability to be in control of how much alcohol they drink, they are still self-destructive, and a danger to themselves and others.

Some of the common signs and symptoms of alcohol abuse include:

- ❖ Repeatedly neglecting your duties at home, at work or at school when drinking.
- ❖ Using alcohol while operating equipment, driving, or taking medication.

- ❖ Consistently getting into trouble with the law while drinking
- ❖ Drinking at the risk of destroying relationships
- ❖ Using drinking to relax or de-stress

The risk of becoming a full-blown alcoholic is huge, and varies depending on the difficulty of certain situations. It will sneak up on you as you develop a tolerance for alcohol, and binge drinkers face an even greater risk.

➤ Signs and Symptoms of Alcoholism

Alcoholism is the severest form of problem drinking. It involves all the symptoms of alcohol abuse, but it also involves another element, which is physical dependence. If you rely on alcohol to function, feel as if your body requires it, and find yourself going into withdrawal when you can't get it, you're an alcoholic.

➤ Tolerance

Tolerance can be an early warning sign of alcoholism, and means that, over time, you need more and more alcohol to feel the same effects.

Signs of tolerance are as follows:

Having to drink a lot more than you used to in order to get buzzed or feel relaxed, and the ability to drink more than others without getting drunk

➤ Withdrawal

Withdrawal is a huge red flag, and a definite sign of alcoholism. It follows the abrupt discontinuation of a drug that has the capability of producing physical dependence.

Drinking to relieve or avoid withdrawal symptoms is sign of alcoholism, and once your body gets used to the alcohol and it's taken away, it begins to experience withdrawal symptoms.

They include:

- Anxious
- Trembling
- Perspiring
- Nausea or Queasiness
- Inability to sleep
- Depression
- Agitation
- Tiredness
- Loss of appetite
- Headaches

Some of the more severe and dangerous withdrawal symptoms include hallucinations, confusion, seizures, fever, and agitation.

➢ **Additional Signs and Symptoms of Alcoholism**

- Lack of control with your drinking.
- The inability to quit.
- Other activities suffer because of your drinking.
- Asserting too much energy and focus on alcohol.
- Drinking in spite of the fact that you know it's causing problems.

➢ **Denial**

This is a huge obstacle when it comes to getting help. Your desire to drink overpowers your ability to think rationally, even though you know you're in trouble. It also enhances the troubles that already exist on your job, and at home, and financially and will cause the destruction of all of your relationships.

Smoking Cessation

Causes of Smoking Cessation

➢ **Adults**

Although most people don't really give thought to why or when they smoke, knowing when and why you smoke can be very helpful in choosing a strategy for quitting, that is most likely to work.

Many people smoke:

- ❖ To relieve tension after an argument, while under stress or when feeling angry or depressed.
- ❖ To help control weight issues
- ❖ To help you focus, concentrate or to boost your energy level
- ❖ To feel like you fit in with your friends

➢ **Children and Teens**

Most children and teens smoke cigarettes, cigars, and even smokeless tobacco because their friends are doing it. Many of the movies and TV shows our children watch make smoking seem cool and appealing. Among teens, girls often use smoking as a way to try and control their weight.

Some teens believe smoking makes them look more mature, independent, and self-confident. Some smoke as a way of rebelling against their parents, but have no idea just how addictive cigarettes are. If you have a child that smokes, it may be helpful for you to share with them, some of the reasons why they should quit, and if you currently smoke or have quit smoking, let them know how difficult it cab be to quit. Remember that your child is more likely to smoke if you do, and are also more likely to quit if you do.

➢ **Quitting**

It's difficult to focus on quitting while you're craving tobacco, and it would be helpful to prepare yourself before attempting to quit, by preparing yourself mentally, for a life without a dependence for nicotine.

➢ **Finding reasons to quit**

It is important to understand that quitting smoking for someone else probably won't motivate you to quit, but having your own reasons for quitting will. Think about it, and then ask yourself what are some of the things that would really motivate you to quit.

- ❖ Is it because you want to stay healthy?
- ❖ Do you want to have more control over your life?
- ❖ Are you tired of feeling controlled by tobacco?

Your reasons for quitting may be different from those of a teenager. Talking to them may help them understand the importance of quitting. Talking to your family and friends, can give you the support you need to help you decide to quit.

➢ The risks of smoking

There are many risks in smoking and all of them involve serious health problems.

Short-term risks include:

- ❖ Shortness of breath
- ❖ Asthma
- ❖ Consistent coughing

Long-term risks include:

- ❖ Heart attack
- ❖ Stroke
- ❖ Lung disease
- ❖ Lung cancer

Risks to those who inhale second-hand smoke include:

- ❖ Lung cancer
- ❖ Heart disease
- ❖ SIDS or sudden infant death syndrome
- ❖ Ear infections
- ❖ Asthma

Most of all of the health risk of smoking will go away if you quit.

➢ The rewards of quitting

When quitting smoking you will:

- ❖ Feel better and be able to do more
- ❖ Have less coughing and shortness of breath
- ❖ Look younger
- ❖ Set a good example for others to follow (especially children)
- ❖ Save money
- ❖ Save your teeth
- ❖ Ensure that your breath, hair, clothing, home, vehicle, and children will smell better
- ❖ Be in control of your habit
- ❖ No longer feel embarrassed because you're a smoker

➢ Why you should quit

As a smoker you're probably aware that continuing to smoke is bad for your health, and that if you quit it will reduce the risk of getting a disease that is related to smoking. For smokers, there is a 1 out of 2 chance that they will die 13 to 14 years earlier than they would if they were a non-smoker. Those who quit reduce their risk of getting cancer or having a heart attack, and the sooner they quit the sooner the risks go away.

No matter how old you are you can benefit if you quit smoking and decrease the risk of:

- ❖ An early death
- ❖ Heart attack
- ❖ Stroke
- ❖ Lung cancer
- ❖ Other lung diseases

- ❖ Cancer of the larynx, mouth, throat, esophagus, intestines, bladder, kidney and pancreas
- ❖ Gum disease and loss of teeth
- ❖ Emphysema

Pregnant smokers run the risk of delivering early, and having a baby with a low birth weight.

When you quit smoking you will immediately notice that certain side effects will go away such as: shortness of breath, lack of energy, and asthma symptoms. For each year you go without smoking your lungs will repair themselves more and more. Other benefits to quitting are a reduction in health risks for your family that is due to second-hand smoke.

Contrary to popular opinion, natural, low-tar and low-nicotine cigarettes are no safer than regular ones. So don't be misled by companies trying to sell their products at your expense. In addition, there are also risks to using smokeless tobacco and e-cigarettes.

➢ **Smoking relapse**

If you slip up and smoke a cigarette do not give up. Find someone to talk to who has quit, or talk to a counselor and ask for ideas of what you can do. If taking medicine or using a nicotine replacement, unless you begin smoking on a regular basis again, continue doing what you're doing. Remember, many people who quit for good may try many times before it happens, so you're not alone if you go back to smoking before you finally quit.

➢ **What you may not know**

Under the Affordable Care Act, there are many health insurance plans that will cover preventive care services at no cost to you, which include: checkups, vaccinations and screening tests.

If you have a relapse don't look down on yourself, this is just a sign that a different approach is needed. If you didn't use medicines or a nicotine replacement method, consider doing so the next time. Methods such as gum, patches, medicines and counseling can be more effective, and can even double your chances of success. Think about what made you relapse. It could be that you couldn't handle the cravings, or there wasn't enough support from family and friends, or maybe you were under too much stress. Whatever the reason may be, keep in mind that help is always available when you get ready to try again.

➢ **Staying smoke free**

In order to quit smoking, you must learn how to confront and deal with your craving and the temptation to smoke, but in order to remain smoke-free, you must learn to think and act like a non-smoker.

Some people make it through the first few weeks with no problem, and then find that they run into trouble and go back to smoking, as they go into the 3rd or 4th week and the physical cravings have ceased. Some researchers say staying smoke-free may depend on one's ability to start seeing their self as a non-smoker.

➢ **Tips on how to deal with cravings during the first few weeks**

In the beginning, quitting smoking can cause you to go through changes that don't feel good at all. During withdrawal you will tend to feel irritable, hungry, and anxious. In addition, you could have trouble sleeping, struggle with altering your smoking addiction and even have trouble concentrating, but these symptoms will go away, and especially if you are taking medicine. This may be a lot to handle, but don't give up. In the end you will feel so much better.

The following are tips that can help you during the first few weeks:

❖ Learn how to gain control of your craving and temptations
❖ Don't smoke at all, not even a puff
❖ Avoid the things that trigger smoking such as alcohol and stress
❖ Remove all cigarettes form your home and vehicle
❖ If you do slip up, stay calm, and remember that you have a plan, and remind yourself of how hard you have worked to kick this habit for good

Street and Prescription Drugs

Substance abuse is a medical condition that interferes with one's ability to work, complete school work and family obligations, in addition it also hinders one's ability to maintain relationships with family and friends, and can result in legal problems and unsafe behavior. It can result in an increased amount of substance use, even to the point of using unethical methods to obtain them.

➢ **Understanding Substance Abuse**

The most commonly abused substances are: **Depressants**, **Stimulants**, **Hallucinogenic substances**, and **Opioids**. Athletes have been known to abuse **Anabolic steroids** in order to improve their athletic performance.

- ❖ **Depressants** include substances like alcohol, barbiturates and benzodiazepines.
- ❖ **Stimulants** include substances like amphetamines, cocaine, MDMA or ecstasy.
- ❖ **Hallucinogenic** include substances like LSD or angel dust.
- ❖ **Opioids** include substances like, Oxycodone, which is OxyContin, Hydrocodone, which is Vicodin, Hydrmorphone, which is Dilaudid and Mepridine, which is Demerol.

Substance abuse is a very complex medical problem, and though most people think it's just a matter of having will power when it comes to kicking a drug addiction, that's not really the case, because it actually affects the brain. Because of the stigma that is associated with substance abuse, many health care professionals no longer use terms like addiction and drug addiction, but have resorted to using terms such as, substance use problems.

➢ **Causes of Substance Abuse Problems**

The main chemical messenger that is involved with the brain's reward mechanism is called Dopamine, and pretty much every substance that is associated with substance abuse affects the reward mechanism in the brain. Because the substance makes the user feel good, each time they use, it leaves them wanting more and more, and over a period of time, changes takes place within the brain causing the pleasure that comes from the substance to decrease, and requiring more of it in order to get the same feeling.

There are many factors that play a role in substance abuse, but the actual causes of it are not clear. The risk of substance abuse seems to be higher for those whose family members struggle with substance abuse therefore it would appear that it could be hereditary. Where you live, work and go to school can have an affect on your substance abuse issues, and so can one's family, friends, cultural, and religious beliefs. It can also be affected by mental health issues such as, anxiety and depression, and also when attempting to deal with negative emotions like sadness anger and etc.

> **Symptoms and Complications of Substance Use Problems**

When suffering from substance abuse it can affect you either physically, psychologically, or both.

A **physical dependence** includes developing a tolerance to a substance. This means that you will require more of the drug in order to obtain the same effect. When attempting to break free from substance abuse, people suffer from withdrawal symptoms such as, tremors, headaches, and loose stool. Withdrawing from drug abuse can also be life threatening and even cause mental or psychological problems like depression and anxiety

Just because someone is physically dependent on a substance, it doesn't mean they will be psychologically dependent, and this is especially so if the medication is being used for a real medical problem.

A **psychological dependence** includes feeling as if a substance is required in order to feel good and function properly. With a psychological dependence, you will have a constant craving for the drug or substance, and will do whatever is necessary to get it. When dealing with substances that cause psychological dependence, they usually affect the brain in some way and can also have one or more of the following effects:

- ❖ Analgesia, (feeling no pain)
- ❖ Sedation (drowsiness)
- ❖ Euphoria, (having a high feeling)
- ❖ Respiratory, (shallow or slow breathing)
- ❖ Small eye pupils
- ❖ Itching and flushed or reddened skin
- ❖ Constipation (Bowel blockage)
- ❖ Slurred or unclear speech
- ❖ Confusion or poor judgment
- ❖ Mood changes
- ❖ A lowering of anxiety
- ❖ A feeling of superior abilities
- ❖ An effect on your senses

Some of the many complications that come from substance abuse is as follows: liver, lung and heart disease, vitamin deficiencies and also brain damage. There are also substances that will cause birth defects and others that damage the immune system, therefore increasing the risk of infections.

Those who use amphetamines run the risk of having a heart attack, a stroke, severe anxiety, and also paranoia. Hallucinogens cause people to have hallucinations, distorting their minds, whereby causing them to become temporarily psychotic and try things they can't realistically do, like flying. When sharing dirty needles people run the risk of contracting conditions like AIDS or hepatitis. Another reality is that of having an overdose, which depending on what drug one is using, can even lead to death.

The other complications that may come as a result of substance abuse include, problems at work, with family, and in personal relationships. Those neglecting their family will create problems in the home, with their spouses and children.

There may be times when they will commit criminal acts to support their habit, such as stealing. Many deaths and injuries have occurred as a result of someone driving while under the influence of drugs. There will be times when the substance will affect one's ability to go to work or school, and pregnant women who abuse drugs run the risk of causing their fetus to become addicted to their drug of choice.

➢ Diagnosing Substance Abuse Problems

The evidence of whether or not someone is using substances can be shown through blood and urine tests, however these tests will not reveal if there is a substance abuse problem.

Substance abuse problems may exist if the following occurs:

- You are not able to stop using a substance, or reduce the amount being used.
- You find yourself becoming angry or defensive when someone comments about your use of substances
- You are feeling guilty about your substance use
- You are using a substance soon after getting out of bed

If you believe you or someone you know has a substance abuse issue, it is important that contact your doctor, a local support group or even a community center to seek advice on how to get the assessment necessary, to determine if you need treatment.

➢ Symptoms of Opioid Withdrawal

Long or prolonged use of opioids can cause a person to develop a physical dependence and tolerance, meaning their body requires it, and they need more and more of the narcotic in order to reach the same intended goal. At this point opioid users will usually begin to take more of the drug, so they can continue to get high. If a person becomes addicted to opioids, and attempt to stop taking them, they will begin to experience withdrawal symptoms that include:

- ❖ Anxiety (nervousness)
- ❖ Irritability (touchy or cantankerous)
- ❖ Craving for the drug
- ❖ Rapid breathing
- ❖ Yawning
- ❖ Runny nose
- ❖ Salivation (drooling)
- ❖ Gooseflesh (pimples)
- ❖ Nasal stuffiness
- ❖ Muscle aches
- ❖ Vomiting
- ❖ Abdominal cramping
- ❖ Diarrhea
- ❖ Sweating
- ❖ Confusion
- ❖ Enlarged pupils
- ❖ Tremors (the shakes)
- ❖ Loss of appetite

Although the opioid withdrawal symptoms do not present any medical dangers, they can still be agonizing and unbearable, causing one to continue taking them. Usually the severity of the withdrawal symptoms and how long they last depend upon how long the abuse had been taking place and also how much they were taking.

The symptoms of opioid drug withdrawal aren't medically dangerous. But they can be agonizing and intolerable, contributing to continued use in general, how severe opioid drug withdrawal symptoms are, and how long they last, depends on how long and how much they have been taking the opioids.

In order to successfully rid your self of an opioid addiction, and prevent withdrawal symptoms, a person must go through a process called detoxification or detox. This process consists of taking medicines such as methadone, buprenorphine (sometimes combined with naloxone), and naltrexone, which can be taken in various forms. Once the detox process is completed, the person is free from their addiction, but there could still be a psychological dependence. If stress or other problems that led to the abuse continues to be a part of your daily life, relapse is possible.

> **Treatment and Prevention for Substance Abuse Issues**

Treatment for substance abuse may take a few weeks or even months and relapses is possible, but it is curable and for many, treatment is successful in the long term.

There are a variety of treatment options that are available.

Every plan of treatment depends totally on each individual need, and there are many things that need to be taken into consideration such as:

- ❖ The severity of the problem
- ❖ The support network
- ❖ The desire or motivation to enter into a treatment plan

As the individual needs of the person change, the plan for their treatment may need to be altered.

Possible treatment includes the following:

- ❖ Joining support groups
- ❖ Detoxification
- ❖ Counseling
- ❖ Harm reduction

There are medications available, which can also be used in conjunction with the other types of treatment.

Those dealing with alcohol abuse issues may be given naltrexone, a medication used to help reduce cravings for alcohol. There is also acamprosate, a medicine used to rebalance certain brain chemicals in those suffering from substance abuse.

During the withdrawal or detox process, other medications are sometimes used as a standard procedure, for helping with withdrawal symptoms. There are certain substances that an individual will have to be gradually weaned off of during detox, where they are given lower and lower dosages. In some cases, they may be given less harmful drugs rather than the ones they are addicted to, one example of a drug substitution is giving Methadone, (which is less harmful to the brain), to those addicted to heroin.

No two people are the same, and there are many different reasons why people abuse drugs, alcohol and tobacco, but for sure our society pays a high cost because of it, and it is evident when we look in our hospitals, and emergency departments and see the toll it takes on the health of those that abuse these substances. The connection between drugs and crime is evident when you look at the increase in jail or prison intake. Studies have shown that although finding effective treatment for and prevention of substance abuse is difficult, the best type of national prevention is that of drug education and prevention that is aimed at children and adolescents.

The 2012 National Household survey that was done on drug abuse in the U.S. shows, that 24 million people ages 12 and over use some form of illicit drugs. This same survey estimated that 6.8% of Americans either abuse or are addicted to alcohol, and 22% smoke cigarettes. When these substances are abused they produce some form of intoxication that inevitably alters one's judgment, their perception, hinders their attention span and also the amount of physical control they have.

➢ **Counseling is almost always a part of treatment**

Counseling assists the person in understanding their substance abuse issues and developing effective coping skills.

Treatment programs can vary depending on the region an individual lives in. Some programs require a person to visit a treatment center on a daily, or regular basis, while others involve staying at a treatment facility for a limited amount of time. Services and treatment can vary depending on the program chosen, and also each individual center. Everyone should be comfortable with the treatment plan they enter into.

During the recovery process there is always the possibility of a relapse. Although relapsing doesn't feel good, it is only a temporary setback, and can actually be a learning tool, to help understand what triggers one to use substances, and also how to develop different strategies to help deal with those triggers in the future. It must be understood that while recovery can be a long process for some people, it is very possible to attain, and that though relapse may be disappointing, each one brings you closer to recovery.

There are many different prevention programs available that has proven to help prevent substance abuse issues. Helping our youth understand the risks of substance abuse, by developing open and honest communication within families, will help reduce the risk of them developing substance abuse problems. It is important to discuss drug and alcohol use with your family, and if you are not sure how to communicate the dangers of substance abuse to them, contact your doctor for information and resources.

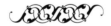

CHAPTER 10

Mental Health Illnesses

Anxiety

Anxiety, also known as a panic attack, is a stress related disorder. It is an overwhelming fear that comes on for a short period of time with no warning, and for no rational reason and it is believed that its causes are very complex.

Some anxiety, such as that experienced by those suffering from Post Traumatic Stress Disorder, stem from trauma, and other life experiences. It is suggested by scientists that anxiety disorders, also stem from a variety of genetic, developmental, environmental and psychological factors as well.

➢ Types of Anxiety Disorders

Anxiety can portray itself in different ways, and the six primary types of anxiety disorder include:

- ❖ Obsessive-compulsive disorder (OCD)
- ❖ Panic Disorder
- ❖ Post-traumatic stress disorder (PTSD)
- ❖ Social anxiety disorder or social phobia
- ❖ Generalized anxiety disorder (GAD)
- ❖ Phobias

Anxiety is a normal reaction to stress, and can be positive. It has the ability to help people cope, however when it becomes excessive, fits no where in a particular situation, or lasts a long time, it can also interfere with your everyday activities and may affect the way you get along with others.

It is important to note that the different types of anxiety disorders have a variety of symptoms. Some may have a series of short-term occurrences of intense fear, while others have overstated worry and tension on a regular basis or in everyday social situations. Anxiety can sometimes develop physical symptoms such as heart pounding, trouble breathing, trembling, sweating, or being easily startled. Many times, anxiety disorders can contain symptoms such as ongoing, unwanted thoughts, or repetitive behavior.

➢ **Generalized anxiety disorder**

You're usually dealing with generalized anxiety disorder if constant worries and fears sidetrack you from your daily duties, or you're constantly struggling with the feeling that something bad is about to happen. People suffering from GAD are restless or anxious much of the time without knowing why, and are often characterized as worrywarts.

➢ **Anxiety attacks (Panic disorder)**

When dealing with anxiety attacks or panic disorder, you will have a continuous influx of unexpected panic attacks coupled with the fear of having another one. This particular anxiety disorder may also be accompanied by agoraphobia, which is characterized as a fear of getting caught up in places where little or no help would be available in the event that a panic attack took place. People with this disorder will most likely avoid things such as airplanes where they would be confined, or shopping malls where there would be an enormous amount of people.

➢ **Obsessive-compulsive disorder**

When dealing with obsessive-compulsive disorder (OCD) you will find yourself confronted with troubling thoughts or behavior with no ability to stop or control them. If you have OCD, you may be plagued by obsessions, such as a repeatedly worrying that you forgot to turn off the stove, or iron or that you might do harm to someone. People with OCD is said to also wash their hands repeatedly.

➢ Phobia

When dealing with a phobia one will have an unrealistic fear of a particular object, activity, or situation that isn't likely to present any danger at all. Some of the most common phobias include fear of animals such as snakes and spiders, and fear of flying and heights. If your phobia is severe enough you could possibly go to great lengths to avoid these things altogether, but this will only serve to give more power to the phobia.

➢ Social anxiety disorder

When dealing with social anxiety disorder, also known as social phobia, this crippling fear will give you a false impression of being viewed negatively by others, and that you will somehow become publicly humiliated. This disorder can be characterized as extreme shyness that will cause you to avoid socializing altogether. The most common type of social phobia is known as performance anxiety or stage fright.

➢ Post-traumatic stress disorder

Post-traumatic stress disorder is very extreme and is commonly triggered as the result of a traumatic or life-threatening event. (PTSD) is characterized as a panic attack that almost never lets up. Some of the symptoms are said to include flashbacks or nightmares about the traumatic event, being overly cautious, very easily startled, isolating oneself, and avoiding any and all circumstances that may remind you of that event.

➢ Signs and symptoms of Anxiety

Whenever someone is faced challenging situations such as a job interview, a tough exam or even a new love relationship, it's normal to feel anxious. But if you find that your worries and fears have begun to overwhelm you and is causing problems in your life from day to day, there is a very good possibility that you may be suffering from an anxiety disorder. There are many types of anxiety disorders, and a gamut of effective treatments and self-help strategies, and once you have a clear understanding of your particular anxiety disorder, you can then begin to take the necessary steps to reduce your symptoms and also re-claim control of your life.

➢ Understanding anxiety disorders

Although many view it as something bad, it is very natural to experience anxiety. In response to danger, it is like an automatic alarm system that goes off whenever you're faced with a threat, any kind of pressure, or a stressful situation. If you allow it to anxiety can be helpful by inciting you to stay alert, focused and motivated when it comes to solving problems. However, one can tell when it ceases to be functional, normal and productive because it will begin to interfere with their daily activities and relationships.

➢ Additional Signs and Symptoms

- ❖ Constantly tense, worried, or edgy
- ❖ Constant interference with work, school, or daily responsibilities
- ❖ Consistently dealing with unusual bouts of fear that is unshakable
- ❖ Difficulty dealing with everyday situations or activities for fear that they will cause problems
- ❖ Unexpected panic attacks or heart-pounding panic
- ❖ Feelings of paranoia

Anxiety disorder is not a single disorder, but instead is a group of related conditions, and for this reason everyone who deals with it will not necessarily act the same.

For example; some may be hit with an anxiety attack without any warning. Someone else might freak out at the thought of mingling with others. Another individual may struggle with an immobilizing fear that keeps them from doing something as simple as driving and flying on a plane, or an uncontrollable passage of disturbing thoughts.

Though different, all anxiety disorders share a major symptom: living with persistent fear or worry when dealing with situations that the average person is not threatened by.

> **Emotional symptoms of anxiety**

In addition to the main symptoms of anxiety, the following list consists of some other everyday emotional symptoms

- Feelings of uneasiness or concern
- The inability to concentrate
- Feeling stressful and nervous
- Expecting the worst
- Being touchy
- Impatience
- On a constant search for signs of danger
- Feelings of absentmindedness

> **Anxiety attacks and their symptoms**

Anxiety attacks are also known as panic attacks and are episodes of intense panic or fear. Although they usually occur suddenly, and without warning, there is sometimes an obvious trigger. Some of those triggers can be getting stuck in an elevator, being in a car for many hours, starting a new job or concentrating on a paper you have to write. In other cases, the attacks come in a spur of the moment.

These attacks usually climax within ten minutes, and rarely last over thirty. But despite the fact that it's a short period of time, the fear that one experiences can be just as severe as if they're about to take their last breath or lose complete control. The physical symptoms of anxiety attacks are so frightening that many people have been convinced that they're having a heart attack. Each attack heightens the fear of having another one and especially out in the public where there is no escape.

> **Symptoms of anxiety attacks include but are not limited to:**

- Overwhelming fear
- Thoughts of losing your mind

- ❖ Pounding heart
- ❖ Feeling like you'll pass out
- ❖ Inability to breathe
- ❖ Chills
- ❖ Vomiting
- ❖ Trembling
- ❖ Becoming isolated

> **Self-help for anxiety disorders and attacks**

Anxiety is a part of life, and the fact that one is anxious does not mean they have an anxiety disorder. Anxiety can be brought on by a number of different things; from your work schedule, a lack of sleep, pressure at home, or even too much caffeine.

The unhealthier and stressful, you are the more likely you are to feel anxious, however if you feel you like you worry too much, discovering whether or not you have an anxiety disorder may be as simple as doing an evaluation of how well you take care of yourself. For example:

- ❖ How often do you relax?
- ❖ Do you have an outlet for your stress?
- ❖ Are your healthy?
- ❖ Are you weighted down with responsibilities?
- ❖ Do you keep your problems locked up inside?
- ❖ Do you eat right?
- ❖ Do you sleep enough?

If you find yourself stressed, make a list of things you can do to bring your stress level back down. It's okay to delegate responsibility, or share what you're going through with a friend or loved one. Venting can be healthy, and you'll be surprised at how much relief you may feel. Take a weekend and go away by yourself. There are many things you can do to de-stress.

- **Other activities that may be helpful include:**
  - Writing down your worries during your anxiety attack. This will keep you busy and possibly shift your mind away from negative thoughts.
  - Nothing in life is set in stone, and no one can predict what may happen from day to day. Learn to accept the fact that life is uncertain, and don't pressure yourself to always try to have a ready solution to every troublesome situation.
  - Learn different techniques that will help you relax, such as meditation and deep breathing.
  - Adopt good eating habits. Begin your day by eating a good breakfast, and learn to incorporate more fruit, vegetables, grain, and protein for energy.
  - Smoking and drinking will only cause an increase in anxiety, and neither is healthy.
  - Make sure you incorporate a good exercise regime into your schedule. Exercise can help you feel better both physically and emotionally.
  - Sleep is important. When you don't get a proper amount, which is usually around 8 to 9 hours, it can intensify your anxiety.

- **When to seek professional help**

Self-help techniques can be very helpful, but if you find yourself becoming overwhelmed with worry, or your anxiety attacks are increasing and interrupting your life, it's probably time to seek out professional help. It is also helpful to visit your primary care physician to make sure your anxiety is not being brought on by an underlying medical condition, recreational drugs, prescription drugs, over the counter medicines, or supplements.

There are two types of behavior therapy used to treat anxiety disorders, and they are cognitive-behavioral therapy, and exposure therapy. Instead of centering attention around psychological struggles or past problems they focus on behavior. In general, this therapy can take anywhere between 5 and 20 weekly sessions.

➢ **Cognitive-behavior therapy**

This type of therapy will assist you in recognizing and also confronting negative thought patterns as well as illogical views that help feed your anxiety.

➢ **Exposure therapy**

This type of therapy will help persuade you to face your fears while in a safe, controlled atmosphere. By repeatedly exposing you to the objects, or situations that causes your fears, you will begin to develop an increased sense of control. And little by little your anxiety will vanish once you see that no harm will come to you.

Bipolar Disorder

➢ **What is Bipolar Depression disorder?**

Bipolar disorder, also known as manic depressive or manic depression, is a serious mental illness marked by alternating periods of elation and depression. It's a disorder that can lead to risky behavior, damaged relationships and careers, and even suicidal tendencies if it's not treated.

➢ **Signs and symptoms of bipolar disorder**

When it comes to bipolar disorder it can affect different people differently, and this is because the symptoms consist of such a wide range of patterns, harshness, and frequency. There are those who lean more towards either mania or depression, and then there are those who float back and forth equally between the two. Some people's moods are interrupted on a regular basis, and then others only have a few occurrences throughout their entire life.

➢ **Bipolar Disorder Causes**

There is no single cause for Bipolar Disorder. It seems that some people develop bipolar disorder genetically, however, everyone that has an inherited weakness doesn't develop the illness. This indicates that there are other causes other than genes. Brain imaging reports have shown physical fluctuations in the brains of people who have Bipolar Disorder. Other research has suggested that it could be caused by neurotransmitter imbalances, abnormal thyroid function, circadian rhythm disturbances, and high levels of the stress hormone cortisol.

It is believed that external environmental and psychological factors are also responsible for the development of Bipolar Disorder. These external issues are known as triggers. Triggers have the potential to initiate new occurrences of mania or depression or make current symptoms worse, but many occurrences develop without any obvious trigger.

> **Bipolar Disorder Triggers**

- **Stress**

    If someone has a genetic weakness, and they experience a stressful life event this can trigger Bipolar Disorder. The events that will trigger Bipolar Disorder usually include severe or sudden changes, which can be either good or bad. These are events such as getting married, going away to school, losing a loved one, losing a job, or moving.

- **Substance Abuse**

    Substance abuse isn't a cause of bipolar disorder, but it has the potential to ignite an occurrence and make the progression of the disease worse. Drugs like cocaine, ecstasy, and amphetamines have the ability to trigger mania, and likewise alcohol and tranquilizers have the ability to trigger depression.

- Medication

    The medications that have the greatest tendency to trigger mania is antidepressant drugs. There are other meds that may cause mania also, and they consist of over-the-counter cold medicines, appetite suppressants, caffeine, corticosteroids, and also thyroid medication.

- ❖ **Seasonal Changes**

  Seasonal patterns often trigger occurrences of mania and depression. The most common season for manic occurrences is summer, and the most common seasons for depressive occurrences are fall, winter, and spring.

- ❖ **Sleep Deprivation**

  Sleep is critical for those suffering from bipolar disorder, and even by skipping just a few hours of rest you can trigger an occurrence of mania.

➤ **Types of Mood Interruptions or Disturbances**

There are four different types of mood interruptions that make up bipolar disorder which include mania, hypomania, depression, and mixed episodes, and each one has a very distinct set of symptoms.

➤ **Mania**

When it comes to the manic stage of bipolar disorder, there are common sensations that are experienced such as intensified energy, inspiration or creativity, and jubilance. Those experiencing a manic occurrence usually talk non-stop, get very little sleep, and are very energetic. They can also feel like there's nothing they can't accomplish, and that they're unbeatable, or created to do great things.

But though mania may feel good in the beginning, it will eventually escalate to a point where they lose control. During a manic occurrence people tend to behave recklessly, which can result in things such as: gambling away their savings, being promiscuous, or making grave business decisions. They have also been known to showcase their anger, and act very irritable and violent. They are prone to provoke others, act out when people don't agree with them, and pointing the finger at anyone who speaks out against their behavior. Some even get to a point where they begin hearing voices.

➤ **Hypomania symptoms**

Hypomania is not as severe as mania. Those struggling with a hypomanic condition usually feel, jubilant, full of energy, and very productive, but they have the ability to continue on with their daily activities, never losing touch with reality. To those who aren't aware of the condition it may seem as if this person is just in a very good mood. But, hypomania can also result in them making bad decisions that will harm their relationships, jobs or careers, and statuses. In addition, hypomania can very easily turn into full-blown mania.

- **Common signs and symptoms of mania include:**
  - Feeling up one moment and down the next
  - Impractical, and magnificent views about their capabilities or abilities
  - Getting very little sleep, while feeling extremely energetic
  - Talking a mile, a minute
  - Having your thoughts all over the place; jumping back and forth from one idea to the next
  - Unable to focus or concentrate on one specific thought
  - Clouded judgment and very spontaneous
  - Making reckless decisions without considering the consequences
  - Having both delusions and hallucinations (in severe cases)

- **Bipolar Depression**

In the past, bipolar depression has been confused with regular depression, but research has shown that there are noteworthy variances between the two. This is especially so when it comes to recommended treatments. Most people possessing bipolar depression show no progress while using antidepressants. In fact, one of the risk factors of using antidepressants to treat bipolar depression is that they can make it worse, by triggering mania or hypomania, causing mood conditions to shift quickly, or delaying the progress of other mood stabilizing meds.

Despite how similar they are; certain symptoms are more prevalent in bipolar depression than regular depression. For example, bipolar depression will most likely cause agitation, remorse, random mood fluctuations, and anxiety. In addition, those with bipolar depression also have a tendency to move and speak at a slow pace, sleep obsessively, and also put on weight. Also, they have a greater chance of developing psychotic depression, which is a condition that is characterized by being detached from reality, and experiencing major disability in work and social performance.

➢ **Common symptoms of bipolar depression include:**
  ❖ Feelings of hopelessness, sadness, or emptiness.
  ❖ Irritability and agitation
  ❖ No sense of pleasure
  ❖ Tired or lack of energy
  ❖ Physically and mentally fatigue
  ❖ Loss of appetite and weight change
  ❖ Problems sleeping
  ❖ Problems with memory and concentration
  ❖ Feeling worthless and guilty
  ❖ Having suicidal or death thoughts

➢ **Mixed Episode**

A mixed occurrence shows symptoms of mania or both hypomania and depression. Symptoms of a mixed occurrence include depression mixed with, irritability, anxiety, insomnia, being easily distracted, and thoughts racing through the mind. This mixture of high energy and low mood opens the door to an exceptionally high risk of suicide.

➢ **Bipolar disorder and suicide**

The depressive phase of bipolar disorder is usually quite severe, and chances for suicide is a major risk factor. As a matter of fact, people who suffer from bipolar disorder will usually attempt suicide before those suffering from regular depression, and their suicide attempts are usually more deadly.

For people with bipolar disorder who have regular depressive occurrences, mixed occurrences, along with a history of alcohol or drug abuse, a history of suicide throughout the family, or early signs of the disease there is an even higher risk of suicide.

- **The warning signs of suicide include:**
  - Talking about death, harming their self, or suicide
  - Having feelings of hopelessness or helplessness
  - Having feelings of worthlessness or feeling like a burden to others
  - Doing things that put their life in danger
  - Making funeral arrangements or saying goodbye
  - A sudden interest in purchasing a weapon or trying to get a hold of pills that can kill you.

Suicide talk or threats of suicide should always be taken very seriously. If you or someone you care about is suicidal, call the National Suicide Prevention Lifeline in the U.S. at 1-800-273-TALK **or visit IASP or visit Suicide.org to find a helpline in your country.**

- **Treatment for bipolar disorder**

If you or someone you know has any of these symptoms don't wait to get help. Ignoring the problem will not make it go away, but will most assuredly make it worse. If left untreated Bipolar Disorder will affect every area of your life, but an early diagnosis can prevent these difficulties. The feelings you get when having a manic occurrence may feel good because of the energy and euphoria, but keep in mind that mania and hypomania can be very destructive for you and everyone you love.

- **Basics treatment**

This disorder is chronic and those who have it have been known to relapse. Treatment is important to prevent new occurrences, and should be continued no matter how well you feel.

Treatment through medication alone is not ample enough to fully control bipolar disorder, and in order for treatment to be effective it must consist of medication, therapy, a change of lifestyle, and moral support.

Because of the complexity of this condition, the difficulty of treatment, and the need to closely monitor the medication, the safest thing to do is seek professional psychiatric help.

> **Self-help techniques**

While professional help is a must, there are also self-help methods that can be used in conjunction with medication, and therapy so that you can successfully manage bipolar disorder. Among the smart choices you can make to keep your mood under control, a life style change, and a change in daily habits are a must.

❖ Education

Additionally, it is important to become as educated as possible about bipolar disorder. The more information you obtain, the greater your odds are of being able to assist with your recovery.

❖ Stress relief

It is important to maintain a healthy stress level. Some techniques that would be helpful is avoiding stressful situations, maintaining a stable and healthy work-life, and also different measures of relaxation, such as meditation, deep breathing and cardio exercise.

❖ Support

Support is key for recovery. Support groups can be very helpful, but if you don't feel comfortable reaching out to a stranger, then talk to someone you can trust. This is not a sign of weakness, and while you may view yourself as a burden, those who love you would embrace you and really appreciate your reaching out to them at a time like this.

❖ Healthy Choices

If you feel good chances are your mood won't fluctuate back and forth, reaching this goal is as simple as getting a proper amount of sleep on a regular basis which is particularly important, developing good eating habits, and maintaining healthy exercise habits.

❖ **Monitoring your mood**

In order to prevent another occurrence, it is important that you monitor your symptoms closely, and note any changes in your mood

Depression

Depression is more than the average sadness and mood downswings that people experience throughout life. However, when experiencing these feelings people often use the term depression to describe them. It is a mood disorder that causes persistent feelings of sadness and loss of interest. This condition can affect how you rationalize things, your behavior, and can lead to various emotional and physical issues.

There are different expressions that are used to describe depression, and among them are living in a black hole, and feelings of impending doom. Not everyone that goes into depression experiences feelings of sadness, but instead many feel lifeless, empty, uninterested, angry, hostile and agitated.

The periods of sadness that the average person goes through, is totally different from depression. Depression is like a deep hole that opens up and swallows up the life that you know. It affects one's ability to work, study, sleep, eat and enjoy recreation. In addition, you will experience periods of helplessness, hopelessness, and even insignificance and these feelings can be very intense, offering little or no relief at all.

➢ **Causes of depression**

With depression there are a variety of factors that play a part in terms of the cause of depression. These factors include:

❖ **Biological differences**

Many people suffer with depression due to biological differences seem to have physical fluctuations in their brain, however the implications of these changes are not certain, but could potentially help identify causes.

❖ **Brain chemistry**

In brain chemistry, there are neurotransmitters, which are naturally occurring brain chemicals. These neurotransmitters carry communication between nerves, and could possibly be associated with the cause of depression, when out of balance.

❖ **Hormones**

When the natural balance of the body's hormones change this could cause depression, and may also result in conditions such as thyroid problems, menopause or many other conditions.

❖ **Inherited traits**

Because depression seem to be more common in people who have biological relatives that also suffer from it, researchers are doing studies to find out if genes might play a role in the cause of this condition.

❖ **Life events**

When suffering trauma this can also trigger depression. Some of the tragic events that can cause this condition are, death, or loss of a loved one, highly stressful situations, problems with finances and painful childhood experiences.

➢ **Signs and Symptoms of Depression**

Although depression can vary from person to person, there are some signs and symptoms that are common. You must maintain an awareness of the fact that, even though these symptoms are generally downswings that are associated with life's everyday situations, if you find that you are having more symptoms, that they're stronger, and tend to last longer, it is very likely that you are suffering from depression. If this is the case and the symptoms become too much for you to handle, it is time to seek professional help. Signs and symptoms include:

❖ **Feelings of helplessness and hopelessness**

Having a dreary outlook on life, believing that things will never get better, no matter what you do

❖ **Loss of interest in daily activities**

A complete lack of interest in the things that once brought you joy, and pleasure.

❖ **Changes in weight and appetite**

A significant increase or decrease in weight of more than 5% of per month.

❖ **Sleep changes**

Having a change in sleeping patterns such as insomnia, which interferes with your ability to sleep, or oversleeping.

❖ **Angry or irritable**

Having feelings of irritation, or restlessness, and resorting to violence. Finding that you have a low tolerance level, a short temper, and that everything and everyone seem to work your nerves.

❖ **Having no energy**

Feeling totally drained, tired, and lazy. Feeling like you're carrying an excessive amount of weight although you're not, and that even the smallest or most menial tasks wear you out and take longer to finish.

❖ **Self-loathing**

Hating yourself, feeling as if you are totally worthless, or being severely critical of yourself and finding fault in almost everything you do.

❖ **Behaving recklessly**

Doing things that put your life in danger such as, engaging in activities of drug and alcohol abuse, gambling compulsively, exceeding safe speed limits while driving, or participating in potentially deadly sports.

❖ **Concentration problems**

Having an inability to focus, make the smallest decisions, and also suffering from memory loss.

❖ **Mysterious aches and pains**

   A sudden unexplainable increase in bodily pain such as, headaches, muscle aches, back pain and also pain in the abdomen.

Understanding the Effects of Depression

➢ **Men and depression**

Many view depression as episodes of extreme emotionalism, associating it with a sign of weakness. When dealing with depression men have a tendency to conceal feelings of self-hatred and hopelessness, and are more apt to complain about being tired and irritable, having problems sleeping and a loss of interest as it relates to their hobbies and work. However, when it comes to depression in men their behavior will be marked with anger, hostility, acts of violence, reckless behavior, and substance abuse. They also have a higher rate of suicide than women who deal with depression.

➢ **Women and depression**

Women are more likely to suffer with depression than men. In fact, they are 2 times more likely, and this is partly because of hormonal issues, and can result in the following conditions. Premenstrual syndrome or PMS, which is caused by a change in hormones during the menstrual cycle. It is during this period that women experience bloating, agitation, fatigue and emotional oversensitivity. Premenstrual dysphoric disorder or PMDD, postpartum depression, a condition that many new mothers experience, which is partly due to hormonal changes, and is also known as the "baby blues." Although it is a normal reaction after giving birth, some women plunge into a deep depression. And then there is perimenopause, which sets the stage to enter into menopause because of rapidly changing reproductive hormones. Unlike men, women are more prone to experience guilt, excessive sleeping, overeating, and weight gain. In addition, women are susceptible to depression after experiencing chronic illnesses, injuries, or disability, and also when engaging in crash diets or attempting to quit smoking.

➢ Teens and depression

Some teens seem sad when suffering from depression while others don't. They are normally irritable, hostile, grouchy, and can easily lose their temper. In addition, teens are prone to experience mysterious aches and pain. In teens, if this condition is ignored, it has a tendency to affect them in school, and can also lead to substance abuse, self-hatred and unfortunately homicidal tendencies and suicide. The advantage teens have is that for them depression is highly treatable.

➢ Elderly adults and depression

In older adults the cause of depression includes: loss of independence, loss of a spouse or other loved one, and health issues. This is especially so for those who lack a strong support group. Older adults lean more towards voicing concerns about the physical symptoms than the emotional ones. It is because of this that the problem can go unnoticed. It is highly important for them to receive treatment because of a higher risk of poor health, a high mortality rate and also a higher suicide rate.

➢ Types of depression

It is important to understand what type of depression you are dealing with so you can receive the proper treatment, but it is also important to know that various types have their own unique set of symptoms, causes and effects. The different types are Major Depression and Dysthymia.

❖ Major depression

Major depression totally hinders your ability to enjoy life and experience joy. The symptoms almost never cease and can range anywhere from moderate to severe, typically depression lasts around six months. With Major Depression one can experience one occurrence in their lifetime, but it generally consists of reoccurring episodes.

❖ Dysthymia (recurrent, mild depression)

This condition is considered to be a chronic low-grade type of depression. You will have short periods of a typical mood, but more often than not you will experience mild or discreet bouts of depression. Although the symptoms are milder than those of major depression they can last up to two years, making it extremely hard to enjoy life. Dysthymia also has the ability to produce a condition known as double depression when coupled with major depression. It can weave its way into your personality, giving the feeling that your life has always been this way and that this is just a part of your character. The good news is that even if your symptoms are not treated for a long because they were unrecognizable there is still hope of treating it.

➢ **Treatment**

Depression doesn't affect everyone the same and there isn't just one particular type of treatment. Your best option is to learn as much as you can about your condition and then find out which treatment is best for you.

➢ **Treatment tips:**

❖ **Learn as much as you can**

Because the medical condition must be treated first, it is important to establish whether or not your condition is due to an underlying medical condition.

❖ **The right treatment takes time to find**

Don't expect to find the correct form of treatment over night because it is trial and error and may take some time to pinpoint which treatment is right for you.

❖ **Medications alone is not a cure all**

Although a particular medicine may work well for you, it may not necessarily be appropriate for long-term use. There are other treatments such as therapy and exercise.

❖ **Get social support**

Remember that having a social network consisting of people who not only love you, but of people who are also positive, and motivating and someone you can trust.

- **Time and commitment**

Keep in mind that treatment takes time, and though it may be frustrating and prolonging it is important to understand that this is normal. There will be ups and downs but do not give up.

Lifestyle changes can be very powerful even though they seem simple, and may just be all that is required for you. Even if you need other treatment it is still very important to make the necessary lifestyle changes.

- **Lifestyle changes needed to treat depression**
  - Proper Exercise
  - Good Proper Nutrition
  - Proper amount of Sleep
  - Good Social support
  - Stress reduction

- **Ruling out medical causes**

It is important to be sure that your depression is not a result of an underlying medical condition. If it is therapy, and other treatment will be of little or no help at all, because the depression cannot be properly treated until your doctor is able to determine what the medical condition is and treat it.

Two medical conditions that could potentially mimic depression are:

Hypothyroidism also known as an underactive thyroid. This condition is known to cause mood swings, and especially so in women. If you are taking a lot of different medications, the interaction of certain drugs can also cause symptoms of depression to show up.

- **Therapy**

Of the many types of therapy the three that are most common are: Cognitive behavioral therapy, interpersonal therapy, and psychodynamic therapy. Much of the time these therapy treatments are combined.

Various therapy techniques are used to help you gain knowledge, of how to restructure negative thought patterns, and overcome depression through the use of behavioral skills. Therapy can also help you to understand why you have certain feelings, and figure out what triggers depression in you. In doing so you will also be able to understand the root cause of your depression, and how to stay healthy.

Therapy does for those struggling with depression, what glasses do for those with poor vision. It helps ease the overwhelming sensations, but also allows you to stand back and regain your focus, while helping you to visualize the factors that contribute to your depression.

Some of the areas therapy can help with include:

- ❖ Relationships
- ❖ Setting healthy boundaries
- ❖ Handling life's problems

➢ **Individual and group therapy**

Usually one might think therapy consists of one-on-one sessions, but group therapy can be just as beneficial in treating depression.

There are great benefits with both types of therapy and are as follows:

- ❖ Both normally last an hour
- ❖ Individual therapy helps you to develop strong one-on-one relationships where you feel comfortable talking to someone you don't know about things that are personal and sensitive, and you don't have to share your time with other individuals
- ❖ In group therapy, having the opportunity to hear others share their struggles, allows you to know that you're not going through it alone, and that recovery is possible. This helps to build your confidence, and may give you tips on how to conquer a certain area that you struggle with. This scenario can also inspire you and help you meet and socialize with people that you can identify with but wouldn't have otherwise met.

When in therapy it is important to remember that it could potentially get worse before it gets better, because you're touching on sensitive areas, and that your recovery depends heavily on your ability to be honest with your therapist. Also keep in mind that if you find that you can't connect with your therapist, there are other options available to you.

➢ **Treating with medicine**

If you are being treated with medication, keep in mind that a combination of both therapy and a change of lifestyle can help make your recovery time shorter.

Eating Disorder
Anorexia Nervosa

As humans we all have something about ourselves that we wish we could change, and it's natural, but when you become preoccupied with being thin to the point that it takes over your eating habits, your thoughts and your life, this is a sign that an eating disorder exists. With anorexia, your desire to lose weight becomes more important to you than anything else, along with even losing the ability to see yourself as the beautiful human being that you truly are.

Anorexia is a very serious eating disorder, and it affects both men ad women of all ages. It has the ability to damage your health and is a threat to your life. Just know that you're not alone, and when you get ready to make a change, help is available for you. Treatment will help you feel better, and find the happiness you deserve, as you learn to value yourself.

➢ **What is Anorexia Nervosa?**

It is a very complex eating disorder that has three key features and they are:

- ❖ Refusing to maintain a healthy body weight
- ❖ Developing a great fear of gaining weight
- ❖ Having an inaccurate image of your body

Since you fear becoming fat and are sickened with what your body looks like, eating and mealtimes can become very stressful for you, and all you can do is think about what you can and cannot eat. Your entire day is filled with thoughts of dieting, food and what your body looks like, and this leaves very little time for family, friends and the activities you once loved. Your life becomes one big journey of trying to stay thin and taking extreme measures to do so, and no matter how thin you become, in your mind it's never enough. Even though those who have this problem often deny having an eating disorder, anorexia is indeed a serious and deadly eating disorder. But the good news is that there is hope, and recovery is possible. If the proper treatment along with a support group is received, you or the one you care about will have the ability to break free of the self-destructive patterns of anorexia and regain good health and self-confidence.

➢ Types of anorexia nervosa

There are two different types of anorexia nervosa and they are:

- ❖ The restricting type
- ❖ The purging type

With the restricted type the weight lose goal is achieved by restricting calories in the following ways:

- ❖ Extreme diets
- ❖ Fasting
- ❖ Excessive exercising

With the purging type the weight loss goal is achieved in the following ways:

- ❖ Vomiting
- ❖ Laxatives
- ❖ Diuretics

➢ Questions you can ask yourself to see if you're anorexic

- ❖ Do you feel as if you're fat even though everyone tells you you're not?
- ❖ Do you have a paralyzing fear of gaining weight?

- ❖ Do you feel a need to lie about how much food you eat or hide your eating habits?
- ❖ Have your family and friends become concerned about your weight loss, your eating habits or your appearance?
- ❖ Do you go on a diet, exercise compulsively or take laxatives when you begin feeling overwhelmed or bad about how you look?
- ❖ Do you feel like you're in control of your situation when you don't eat, over indulge in exercise or eat laxatives?
- ❖ Do you base your worthiness on how much you weigh or the size of your body?

➢ **Anorexia Nervosa is not based on one's weight or food**

Many don't realize it but eating disorders are much more complicated than they seem, and the root cause of anorexia really has nothing to do with food and weight, it is simply symptoms of something that is much greater that no amount of dieting can cure such as:

- ❖ Depression
- ❖ Loneliness
- ❖ Insecurity
- ❖ Pressure to be perfect
- ❖ Feeling out of control

➢ **What is the need in your life that anorexia meets?**

It is important for you to understand that anorexia meets a specific need in your life, for example, you may feel helpless in many areas of your life, however you have power over what you eat. The ability to say "no" to food, overcoming feelings of hunger, and having control over how much you weigh may give you feelings of strength and success, at least this is the case for a little while anyway. There may even be a point where you enjoy feeling your hunger pangs, as a reminder of being able to achieve something that most people can't.

You may also be using anorexia as a way of distracting yourself from some difficult emotions you're dealing with. And you feel that if you spend most of your time concentrating on food, dieting and how much you weigh, you won't have to confront the other problems in your life or cope with emotions that are hard to understand. The unfortunate thing is that and thrill you get from starvation or weight loss is very short-lived. Dieting and weight loss does not have the ability to heal the negative image you have of yourself. The only way to deal with the true issue is to identify the emotional need that starving yourself seems to fulfill and find another solution to dealing with it.

> **Signs and symptoms of anorexia nervosa**

When you have anorexia, this means you have to live your life constantly concealing your habits, which makes it difficult in the beginning stages for your family and friends to detect the warning signs. As you are confronted about how you eat, you may try to explain away your chaotic eating habits and reassure any concerns people may have, but as the eating disorder grows worse, those who are close to you will be able to see that a problem exists, and so will you. As anorexia progresses you will become more and more worried about how much you weigh, how you look and what you can and can't afford to eat.

> **The food behavior signs and symptoms associated with anorexia**
>> ❖ **Dieting even though you are thin**

   Going on very strict diets, limiting yourself to certain low-calorie foods and cutting all carbohydrates and fats out of your diet.

>> ❖ **An obsession with calorie counting, amount of fat grams and nutrition**

   You have begun to check all food labels, measure and weigh all of your food portions, keep a journal of everything you eat and purchase books on dieting.

>> ❖ **Not eating at all or lying about what you eat**

   Concealing, playing with or tossing out your food so you won't have to eat, and making excuses to avoid eating

- ❖ **Obsessed with food**

  All you do is think about food, preparing meals for others, collecting recipes, purchasing food magazines, or planning meals but almost never eating anything.

- ❖ **Odd or private food customs**

  Declining to eat in public restaurants, developing firm customs for eating (e.g. cutting food into specific sizes, chewing your food but never swallowing it, and having a special plate to eat on).

➢ **Signs and symptoms of the appearance and body image of an anorexic**

- ❖ **Dramatic weight loss**

  Losing a lot of weight without being ill

- ❖ **Feeling overweight even though you're underweight**

  You feel as if you're overweight in specific areas such as the stomach, hips, or thighs

- ❖ **Obsessed with how you look**

  Totally consumed with your weight, shape of body, or size of clothing. Weighing too much, and worrying about the smallest amount of weight gain.

- ❖ **Very critical of your appearance**

  Spending too much time in the mirror checking for imperfections, finding the smallest things to complain about, never small enough.

- ❖ **Denying that you're underweight**

  You claim you don't have a problem even though you're severely underweight, trying to conceal your body size with baggy clothing.

➢ **Signs and symptoms of purging or cleansing**

- ❖ **Taking diet pills, fat burners, laxatives or water pills**

  You have begun to misuse water pills, diet pills and other products used to lose weight

- ❖ **Deliberately vomiting after eating**

    Excusing yourself from the table quite often during meals to go to the bathroom. Running water to cover up the sound of vomiting or your breath smells like mouthwash or mints.

- ❖ **Suddenly obsessed with exercising**

    Exercising even to the point of injury, through sickness and even bad weather conditions. Under a grueling exercise program to burn calories after eating food you consider to be bad for your weight.

➢ **Anorexia nervosa causes and risk factors**

The answers to the cause of anorexia and other eating disorders are not simple at all. This disease is quite confusing and is compiled of a mixture of social, emotional and biological issues. Even though our society's ideal image is one where we should all be thin, and it plays a huge role in causing eating disorders, there are many other factors that contribute as well which includes:

- ❖ Family environment
- ❖ Emotional issues
- ❖ Low self-esteem
- ❖ Traumatic past experiences

➢ **Psychological causes and risk factors for anorexia**

Generally, those with anorexia are the good sons and daughters that are perfectionists, and overachievers, who do what they're told, and are at the top of the class in all that they do. They appear to have it all together, and focus on pleasing others, but all the while, deep down they feel helpless, worthless and incompetent. They view themselves through a harshly critical lens and to them if they're not perfect in every area, they're a total failure.

➢ **Family and social pressures**

In addition, to trying to fit into societies idea of what you should look like, those struggling with anorexia are faced with other family and social pressures that contribute to their condition. Such pressures come from participating in various activities that require them to be slim such as, ballet, modeling, or gymnastics. It also includes those who have parents who are overbearing, control freaks, put great emphasis on how they look, and are also very critical of their children's appearance. Children who go into puberty, experience a relationship breakup, or going off to school can also fall prey to anorexia.

➢ **Biological causes of anorexia**

Researchers claim anorexia may be genetic, and girls who have siblings that are anorexic are 10 to 20 times more likely to develop the disorder than the average person. They also say people with high levels of cortisol, the brain hormone most connected to stress, and a reduced level of serotonin and norepinephrine are more apt to develop anorexia.

➢ **Major factors that put you at risk of developing anorexia nervosa:**
- ❖ Being dissatisfied with your body
- ❖ Becoming a perfectionist
- ❖ Using strict diets
- ❖ Having Low self-esteem
- ❖ Finding it difficult express your feelings
- ❖ Troubled family relationships

➢ **Having a history of physical or sexual abuse**
- ❖ A history of eating disorders within the family

➢ **The effects of anorexia**

When you severely restrict your calorie consumption, and your body is denied the fuel it needs to function, it automatically goes into starvation mode, slowing down to conserve energy. Essentially, your body starts to eat away at itself, and if it's allowed to continue and you lose more body fat, medical problems will start to compile putting your health at risk.

- ➢ **Some physical effects of anorexia include:**
  - ❖ Depression
  - ❖ Low energy levels
  - ❖ Weak memory and problems thinking
  - ❖ Dry, yellowish skin and fragile nails
  - ❖ Slow bowel movements and bloating
  - ❖ Rotting teeth and gum disease
  - ❖ Feeling dizzy and faint with head aches
  - ❖ Fine hair growth on the face and body
- ➢ **Anorexia affects the whole body**
  - ❖ Brain and nerves (can't think right, fear of gaining weight, sad mood, bad memory, fainting and changes in brain chemistry)
  - ❖ Hair get thin and brittle
  - ❖ Heart (low blood pressure, slow heart rate, fluttering or heart failure)
  - ❖ Blood (anemia, and other blood problems
  - ❖ Muscles and joints (weak muscles, swollen joints, fractures, osteoporosis)
  - ❖ Kidneys (kidney stones or failure)
  - ❖ Body fluids (low potassium, magnesium and sodium)
  - ❖ Intestines (constipation and bloating)
  - ❖ Hormones (periods stop, bone loss, problems growing, trouble getting pregnant, higher risk of miscarriage, C-section, low birth rate and post partum depression)
  - ❖ Skin (bruises easily, dry skin, fine hair growth on body and face)

Healing the Hurts of Yesterday

➢ **Getting help**

It is common to feel as if anorexia is you're your friend or part of your identity, and it's not an easy deciding to get help. Although it feels like anorexia is impossible to overcome, while it may be hard, it's not impossible.

➢ **Steps to recovery**

❖ **Admitting you have a problem**

The initial step to recovery is admitting that your quest to get thinner is out of control, and coming to grips with the fact that it has caused you some physical and emotional damage.

❖ **Talk about it**

Talking about your anorexia can be difficult, especially if you've kept it a secret for a long time. You might feel shame, unsure of yourself, or fearful, but it is vital to understand that you are not in this by yourself. Find someone who will listen and support you as you strive to get better.

❖ **Stay away from people, places, and behaviors that trigger your obsession to lose weight**

Avoid spending time hanging out with friends that indulge in compulsive dieting, and talking about losing weight. In addition, it would be wise to look at magazines and websites that does not promote fitness, fashion, weight loss or anorexia.

❖ **Seek professional counseling**

It is possible to regain your health, learn how to eat naturally and acquire a healthier approach when it comes to your body and the food you eat, but it will require the help of professionals who are trained in giving support and advice about eating disorders.

If you or someone you love has anorexia nervosa, contact the National Eating Disorders Association at 1800-931-2237 for free advice, referrals, and information.

➤ Treatment and therapy

The type of treatment that is best involves a team approach. Anorexia affects both the body and the mind, and proper treatment will require the help of medical doctors, psychologists, counselors, and dieticians. It is important to enlist the participation and support of family members if your treatment is to be successful. Recovery will be much easier if you have a team of people around that you can rely on.

Treatment for anorexia includes three steps and they are:

- ❖ The journey back to a healthy weight
- ❖ Beginning to consume more food
- ❖ Changing how you view yourself and food

➤ Medical treatment

Stabilizing any serious health problems caused by anorexia is always the first priority when starting treatment. If you are so distressed that you want to end your life, or you're so malnourished that your health is in danger, hospitalization may be necessary. This may also be necessary until you reach a weight that is not life threatening. If you're not in immediate danger another option is outpatient treatment.

➤ Nutritional treatment for anorexia

Another element of treatment for anorexia includes nutritional counseling, where you will be taught about proper nutrition, and how to eat healthier by a nutritionist, or a dietician. They will be able to help you come up with and properly follow meal plans that will include a sufficient amount of calories for you to reach and maintain a normal, and healthy weight.

➤ Counseling and therapy

When treating anorexia, it is extremely important to include a module of counseling, so that you can learn to identify the harmful thoughts and emotions that feed your eating disorder, and replace them with more positive views or beliefs. In addition, counseling will help teach you to cope with difficult emotions, problematic relationships, and stressful situations in a more productive way.

> **Overcoming your fears of gaining weight**

It is no easy job to get back to a normal weight, and the very thought of gaining weight will more than likely be very scary. This is especially so if you're being forced into it, and for this reason you may be resistant. But research has proven that as you near the end of your treatment, and get closer to your normal body weight, your chances of recovery will be greater. Therefore, your main goal should be getting to a healthy weight. Talking to other people who have lived with anorexia, or reading up on it, will help you understand that the fear of gaining weight is simply a symptom of anorexia. It will help for you to be honest with your family, and support group about the fears and emotions you're dealing with, so that they will be able to give you the support you need.

> **Helping someone who has anorexia**

One of the most caring, and supportive things you can do is encourage someone who has anorexia to get treatment. But you will need to tread lightly since there is a lot of denial, and defensiveness involved. Telling them that they will die, or showing them articles about how not eating will affect them won't work. Gently expressing your concern, and letting them know you're available to listen is a much better way to approach them. If they are willing to talk to you, just listen, and no matter how out of touch they sound, do not judge them.

Knowing that your child or someone else you love is struggling with anorexia is very upsetting. Although you won't be able to solve the problem on your own, the following are a few ideas you can use, that may help you to make a difference for them.

> **Tips for helping someone with anorexia**
>> ❖ **Think of yourself as being an outsider**

In other words, someone who doesn't have the condition. When you put yourself in this position, there isn't much you can do to solve their problem, because it will ultimately have to be their choice to get help when they're ready to do so.

- ❖ **Become a role model**

    eat right, exercise, and promote a positive body image, and be careful not to make any negative remarks about your body or anyone else's.

- ❖ **Take good care of yourself**

    Even though your friend or family member won't seek advice from a health professional you can, and you can also invite other peers or parents to be a part of the support group.

- ❖ **Don't play the part of the food police**

    Someone suffering from anorexia does not need an authoritative figure standing over them with a calorie counter, they just need compassion, and support.

Avoid making threats, using scare tactics, making angry outbursts and putting them down. It is important to remember that anorexia is often just a symptom of a greater problem such as, extreme emotional distress, and is caused by the person's attempt to cope with emotional pain, stress and/or self-hatred. Making negative comments will do nothing but make it worse.

Binge Eating

Overeating is something that we all do from time to time. At Thanksgiving and Christmas, even though you're already full, you still can't help but to get some dessert. But overeating for binge eater's, is something that is done regularly because of a lack of control. Even though you will feel worse afterwards you overeat, using food to deal with stress and other negative feelings. While it may feel as if you're stuck in an ongoing cycle that seems impossible to escape, the good news is that binge eating is treatable, and with the correct help and support, it is possible to gain control of your eating disorder, and create a healthy relationship with food.

➢ What is binge eating?

Binge eating is an eating disorder that is characterized by an uncontrollable urge to eat, causing people to lose control, and feel powerless to stop eating large amounts of food. The symptoms of binge eating disorder normally develop in the later stages of adolescence or early adulthood. Episodes of binge eating usually lasts about two hours, but many people will binge on and off throughout the day. People who binge often eat whether they're hungry or not, and will still eat long after they are full. Binge eating causes them to overeat as fast as possible, while barely processing what they're eating.

The main characteristics of Binge eating disorder are:

- ❖ Recurrent periods of out of control binge eating
- ❖ Feeling tremendously upset or distraught during or after bingeing

Unlike bulimia there are no attempts to off set binging through vomiting, fasting or over-exercising. People who have a binge eating disorder really want to quit, and because they feel powerless to do so. Therefore, they fight with feeling guilty, disgusted and depressed, worrying about what this disorder will do to their body, while beating themselves up because of their lack of control.

➢ Binge eating cycle

Binge eating leads to weight gain and obesity, which only supports your urge to overeat. It is only comforting for a brief period of time, and after a while the reality that your problems still exists will set in, causing regret and self-hatred. It can be a vicious cycle in the sense that, the worse they feel about themselves and how they look, the more they use food as a means to deal with their emotional issues. It then becomes a repeated cycle: eating to feel better, which makes you feel worse, and then causing you to turn back to food, in an effort to get relief.

➢ Signs and symptoms of binge eating

Binge eating disorder may vary in the sense that it leaves some people overweight, while others maintain a normal weight, but in all cases they will try and conceal their symptoms, and will eat in secret, because they are embarrassed and ashamed of their condition.

- **The behavioral symptoms of binge eating are:**
  - The inability to limit what you eat or quit eating
  - Consuming large amounts of food quickly
  - Continuing to eat even though you're full
  - Concealing or stock up on food so you can eat it later in secret
  - Controlling how you eat in front of others but gorging when you're alone
  - Eating continuously at all times throughout the day with no scheduled mealtimes
- **The emotional symptoms of binge eating are:**
  - Feeling pressure or anxiety that is relieved only by eating
  - Being embarrassed because of how much you eat
  - Feeling like you're numb while binging, as if on auto-pilot
  - Unable to satisfy your hunger
  - Having feelings of guilt, shock, or sadness after binging
  - Feeling desperate to control your weight and how you eat
- **Signs that you have a binge eating disorder**

If you think you might have a binge eating disorder, and after ask yourself the following questions you have more yes answers than no, it is very likely that you have a binge eating disorder.

- Do you feel you're out of control when you're eating?
- Do you always think about food?
- Do you always eat in secret?
- Do you eat until you start feeling sick?
- Do you eat to get away from your troubles, relieve tension, or to comfort yourself?

- ❖ Do you feel sickened or shameful after you eat?
- ❖ Do you lack the ability to stop eating, even though you want to?

➢ **The effects of binge eating disorder**

Binge eating causes many different physical, emotional, and social issues, and those suffering from binge eating disorder have more problems with health, tension, inability to sleep, and thoughts of suicide than those without an eating disorder. Some of the most common side effects of bingeing are depression, anxiety, and substance abuse, but the most noticeable effect is weight gain.

➢ **Binge eating and obesity**

Over a period of time obsessive overeating commonly lead to obesity, and obesity will often lead to numerous health problems which includes:

- ❖ Gallbladder disease
- ❖ Certain kinds of cancer
- ❖ Increased levels of cholesterol
- ❖ Joint and muscle pain
- ❖ A high increase in blood pressure
- ❖ Gastrointestinal issues
- ❖ Heart disease
- ❖ Sleep Apnea
- ❖ Type 2 Diabetes
- ❖ Osteoarthritis

➢ **What causes binge eating?**

There is a combination of different things that cause binge eating disorder and they are: genes, emotions, and life experiences.

➢ **Biological causes**

Biological defects can be a factor for binge eating. Examples are as follows: it could be that the part of the brain controlling the appetite stops transmitting correct signals, that lets you know when you're hungry or full. It has also been shown through research that there is a genetic transformation or change that may cause an addiction to food. Researchers have also found that low levels of a brain chemical known as serotonin may also play a role in obsessive overeating.

➢ **Social and cultural causes**

Two of the things that can set the stage for binge eating and fueling the emotional eating habits of those who struggle with it is, social pressures to be thin, and having parent who use food to console, get rid of, or reward their children. Some other things that can make children vulnerable to binge eating are, being exposed to regular criticism about their bodies, and also being sexually abused as a child.

➢ **Psychological causes**

Depression has been strongly connected with binge eating. Many may struggle with controlling the desire to eat as well as dealing with and expressing how they feel, and have either been depressed before or currently are depressed. Those suffering with low self-esteem, loneliness, and dissatisfaction with their bodies may also struggle with binge eating disorder.

➢ **Binge eating and emotions**

One of the main reasons people binge eat is to deal with negative feelings like stress, sadness, loneliness, fear, and tension, and binge eating can temporarily make these things disappear into thin air, but relief is very short lived. Food can sometimes seem like your only friend, after having a bad day.

➢ **How to stop binge eating**

Binge eating, and food addiction can be difficult to overcome. Unlike other addictions, the drug of choice for you is necessary for your survival therefore it can't be avoided. What you need to do is create a healthier relationship with food, one that is built on meeting your nutritional necessities instead of your emotional ones. If you wish to get rid of your unhealthy eating habits, you must begin eating for health and nutrition which involves creating balanced meal plans, choosing healthy foods when you eat out, and making sure you include the right vitamins and mineral in your diet.

➤ **Ten approaches to overcoming binge eating**

1. Manage stress

   Find ways to deal with your stress and other devastating feelings without using food. Some examples are, meditation, using sensory relaxation techniques, and simple breathing exercising.

2. **Eat three meals everyday along with healthy snacks**

   Start each day with breakfast to help jumpstart your metabolism, and then have a well-balanced lunch and dinner. Don't skip meals to avoid binge eating later in the day.

3. **Avoid all temptation**

   Remove all junk food, and other unhealthy snacks from the house, so you won't be tempted to overeat.

4. **Don't diet**

   Depriving yourself of food, and being hungry from strict dieting can trigger food cravings, and the urge to overeat. Focus on eating in moderation rather than dieting, and find food you enjoy eating that is nutritional, and eat until you are full and not over stuffed. It's okay to keep certain foods around so that you won't develop an even greater craving for them.

5. **Exercise regularly**

   Exercising will not only help with healthy weight loss, but it also helps to get rid of depression, reduces your stress level, and improves your overall health. It boosts your mood and can help put a stop to emotional eating.

6. **Combat boredom**

   If you're bored instead of eating, do something to distract yourself like going for a walk, calling a friend, or start a new hobby.

7. **Make sure you get enough sleep**

   If you're tired, instead of eating to boost your energy level, take a nap or go to bed early.

8. **Listen to your body**

   Learn how to tell the difference between physical hunger, and emotional hunger. If you have recently eaten and your stomach isn't growling, you're not truly hungry, and you should allow the craving time to pass.

9. **Keep a journal of the food you eat**

   Write down what, when, and how much you eat as well as how you feel while you're eating. This will help you discover patterns that may emerge, showing a link between your mood in and your binge eating.

10. **Get the support you need**

    If you don't have a strong support network, you are more likely to give in to binge eating. Talking to someone can help even if it's not a professional. It's okay to look to your family and friends for support, join a support group, and if at all possible talk to a therapist.

➢ **Treatment for binge eating disorder**

Even though you can do a lot of things to help yourself stop binge eating, it is very important to find professional help and treatment. Those who offer professional treatment include: psychiatrists, nutritionists, therapists, and eating disorder and obesity specialists. In order for a treatment program to be successful, it must be directed not only towards your symptoms, but also your damaging eating habits, the root causes of the issue, the emotional triggers that make you want to binge eat, and the problems you have dealing with difficult emotions like stress, worry, fear, and depression. If your life is in danger due to obesity, it may also be very important for you to set a weight loss goal, but since dieting can be a contributing factor for binge eating, your efforts to lose weight need to be monitored by a professional.

➢ **Therapy and for binge eating**

Therapy can be very successful for treating binge eating disorder, and can help you learn how to combat the urge to binge, swap dangerous eating habits for newer healthier ones, keep an eye on what and how you eat as well as your mood swings, and create effective skills that eliminates stress or tension altogether.

There are three types of therapy that are particularly helpful for binge eating disorder, and they are:

❖ **Cognitive-behavioral therapy**

This focuses on bad ideas and behavior that are involved in binge eating. One of the primary objectives of cognitive therapy is to help you gain a greater awareness of how of how you use food to cope with how you feel. It is the therapist's job to help you identify the things that trigger your binge eating and learn how to prevent or overcome them. This type of therapy also involves education on nutrition, healthy weight loss, and different techniques used for relaxation.

❖ **Interpersonal psychotherapy**

This focuses on both issues within a relationship, and interpersonal or social issues that cause obsessive eating. In this case the therapist will assist you in learning how to develop better skills in communication and creating healthier relationships with your family and friends. Learning how to interact better with others, and getting the emotional support you need will help the urge or desire to binge become less frequent and easier to resist.

❖ **Dialectical behavior therapy**

This type of therapy combines both cognitive-behavioral techniques and meditation that helps make your mind clearer or more alert. The importance of therapy is to teach binge eaters how to embrace themselves, be able to endure stress better, and control their emotions. The therapist will also tackle unhealthy attitudes concerning how you eat, how you look, and your weight, and this therapy usually allows access to both weekly treatment and group therapy sessions.

➢ **Support**

It is hard to break the old pattern of binge eating, and from time to time you may slip. This is where both receiving support from your family, friends and therapist and having them come together as a support team will come in handy.

It may also be helpful to join a binge eaters support group, where you can share your experience with others who are compulsive eaters. This can go a long way in helping to reduce the shame and loneliness you might feel. There are many options for choosing a group, including self-help support groups and groups that are more formal.

- ❖ **Group therapy**

    These sessions may cover everything from healthy eating to learning to cope with the desire to binge, and is directed by a trained psychotherapist.

- ❖ **Support groups**

    In this type of session, group members give and receive advice as well as support from one another, and are directed by trained volunteers or health professionals.

➢ **Medications used for binge eating disorder**

It is important to understand that medication is not a cure for binge eating. However, there are some medications that may be used as a comprehensive treatment program, involving therapy, group support and proven self-help methods, that may be useful in helping to treat binge eating disorder.

- ❖ **Topamax**

    Also known as the seizure drug topiramate, this drug may help to decrease binge eating and increasing weight loss. But this drug can be very dangerous, causing side effects such as: Fatigue, dizziness, and burning or tingling sensations.

- ❖ **Antidepressants**

    It has been shown through research that antidepressants may reduce binge eating in those struggling with bulimia, and could possibly help people with binge eating disorder, but studies also show that there are high relapse rates when the drug is discontinued.

➢ Self-prescribing risk

When you self-prescribe any medication, and especially antidepressants, this is very dangerous, and can lead to your death. You should always talk to your primary care physician or mental health professional before you take any medicine.

➢ Helping someone with binge eating disorder

Some of the warning signs that a person is binging are finding heaps of empty food containers and wrappers, cabinets and fridges that have been emptied out, as well as stashes of high-calorie food or junk food that have been hidden away. If you have a loved one or a friend, and you believe they have binge eating disorder, talk to them. It may seem like a discouraging task to start a conversation that is so delicate, and they might deny binging or even become angry and defensive, but they may also welcome the opportunity to talk to someone about their painful ordeal.

They may shut you out at first but don't give up; it might take them a while to admit to having an eating disorder. Keep in mind that even though it may be difficult knowing that someone you love has an eating disorder you can't force anyone to change. The decision to seek help must be theirs. The only help you can offer is in showing compassion, and offering encouragement and support during the course of treatment.

If someone you love has this eating disorder

- ❖ **Encourage them to seek help**
- ❖ **Be supportive**
- ❖ **Avoid insulting and lecturing them and sending them on guilt trips**
- ❖ **Set a good example for them**
- ❖ **Take good care of yourself**
- ❖ **Binge eating disorder treatment and support groups**
- ❖ <u>**Eating Disorder Treatment Finder**</u>- a searchable directory of eating disorder treatment providers, such as doctors, therapists,

dieticians, and support groups. (The something fishy website for eating disorders).

- ❖ **EDreferral.com**
- ❖ **Overeaters Anonymous-** a 12 step program
- ❖ **Eating Disorders Anonymous**

Bulimia Nervosa

Everyone has had times when they have eaten because they were bored, lonely or stressed out. But when it comes to bulimia, overeating is more of an obsession, and rather that eating sensibly to make up for the extra food you've eaten, you discipline yourself by forcefully eliminating waste from your body, fasting, or over exercising to get rid of the extra calories. This back and forward cycle of binging, and then purging yourself affects you both physically, and mentally. With treatment you can get back on track and begin eating healthy again, and learn how to deal with feelings of anxiety, guilt, and shame, which is typically the reason you have the disorder.

> **What is Bulimia?**

Bulimia nervosa, is an eating disorder where you have regular periods of bingeing, followed by panicky efforts to keep from gaining weight, and it effects both men and women of all ages. With bulimia, life becomes a battle that never ends where you're fighting to stay thin, coupled with the overwhelming urge to binge eat. Bingeing isn't something you want to do, but you give in time after time, even though you know it will leave you with feelings of guilt, and shame. On a normal day those who binge will consume 3000 to 5000 calories during one hour. At the end of each binge, you begin to panic and then take drastic measures to undo what you've done by using laxatives, inducing vomiting or over exercising. During this entire process you can feel yourself spiraling out of control.

One important thing to remember is this, what qualifies someone as a bulimic isn't only that they are using laxatives, enemas, vomiting, or water pills to eliminate their food. If you are using excessive exercising, fasting or crash dieting to make up for your binges this also qualifies you as a bulimic.

➢ **How to know if you're bulimic**

When answering the following questions, if you answer yes more than you answer no, you are more than likely bulimic.

- ❖ Are you obsessing over your weight and your appearance?
- ❖ Is your life dominated by food and dieting?
- ❖ Are you afraid you won't be able to stop eating once you start?
- ❖ Do you eat until you get sick?
- ❖ Does eating make you feel guilty, ashamed, or depressed?
- ❖ Do you control your weight by vomiting, or taking laxatives, or diuretics?

➢ **The cycle of bingeing and purging**

The vicious cycle of binge eating, and purging is triggered through dieting, but the interesting thing is that, the stricter your diet, the more apt you are to become worried or even obsessed with food. When your body is starved it respond by strong cravings in an effort to get the nutrition it needs.

When you are overcome by tension, and hunger and your body starts feeling deprived of food, the urge to eat becomes too powerful for you to resist. You might eat food that is forbidden or break a dietary rule that you've put in place, and because you have set your mind to believe it's either all or nothing, as far as you're concerned the slightest slip up is a total failure. You will convince yourself that if you eat a slice of cake, you've already messed up, so you may as well eat the whole thing. The unfortunate thing is that, bingeing is very short-lived, and not long afterward you begin feeling guilty and hating yourself. And then you purge yourself to make up for overeating so that you can regain control again.

The problem with purging is that, it does nothing but boost your desire to binge eat. As you begin a new diet, you may tell yourself this is the last time you'll do it, but in the back of your mind a little voice is reminding you that if you lose control, you can always regain it by vomiting or taking an enema. What you don't understand is that purging is not a cure all, and will never be able to eliminate your desire to binge eat.

➢ **Purging doesn't prevent weight gain**

Although people suffering from bulimia think purging will help them reduce calories, it won't, but what does happen is that, over a period of time they end up gaining weight. The moment you put food in your mouth the body begins to absorb the calories, therefore the most you will eliminate when throwing up immediately after eating is 50% or less of your calorie consumption. Many think taking laxatives and water pills will help them lose weight, but the truth is, they are even less effective. Statistics show that while laxatives only eliminate 10% of the calories you eat, diuretics does nothing at all, and even though you weigh less after taking them, it's only due to a reduction of water not weight loss.

➢ **Signs and symptoms of bulimia**

If you've been struggling with bulimia for some time, you have probably done everything you could think of to hide your purging and bingeing habits. It's natural to feel ashamed about your inability to control yourself when it comes to food, and because of this you probably binge alone. When binge eating, you will do things such as eating a package of cookies, and then replacing them so no one will notice, or shopping at different stores so the clerk won't guess what you're doing, but regardless of how well you keep your secret, those who are closest to you already notice that something is wrong.

➢ **Binge eating signs and symptoms**

❖ **No control over eating**

You can't stop eating, and eat until you are uncomfortable or in physical pain.

❖ **Eating in secret**

You wait until everyone has gone to bed, and then get something to eat so you can eat in private. Going out to get food randomly.

- ❖ **Consuming very large amounts of food**

  You eat a lot but never look bigger

- ❖ **Food is disappearing**

  You hide junk food, and there are a lot of empty food wrappers or containers in the garbage.

- ❖ **You switch back and forth between bingeing and purging**

  You almost never eat normal food portions. You never leave anything on the plate. If you open something you eat all of it in one sitting.

➢ **Purging signs and symptoms**

- ❖ **Making bathroom trips after eating**

  You make a lot of trips to the bathroom during and after meals to throw up, using the sound of running water to cover up the sounds of vomiting

- ❖ **Using water pills, ex-lax, and enemas**

  You purge with diuretics, enemas, or laxatives right after eating. You also take diet pills or try to sweat off pounds using a sauna.

- ❖ **They smell like vomit**

  The person tries to cover up the smell of vomit, by using mouthwash, gum, mints, perfume, or air freshener.

- ❖ **Exercising excessively**

  Does extensive workouts, which include high cardio training, running or aerobics.

➢ **Physical signs and symptoms of bulimia**

- ❖ **Knuckles or hands have scars or calluses**

  You stick your fingers down your throat to induce vomiting

- ❖ **Fat jaw cheeks**

  Because of repeated vomiting

- ❖ **Tooth discoloration**

    Your teeth look yellow, chipped, or clear due to the exposure to stomach acid from vomiting.

- ❖ **Sporadic weight gain or loss**

    Weight fluctuates up and down by 10 lbs. or more because of bingeing and purging.

➢ **Effects of Bulimia**

Bulimia is dangerous for both your body and your life. Dehydration is the most dangerous side effect of bulimia, and this is due to the purging process. Vomiting, laxatives, and water pills can cause dangerously low levels of potassium, through an imbalance of electrolytes. A vast range of symptoms can be triggered by low levels of potassium including, lethargy, cloudy thinking, irregular heartbeat, and even death. In cases where people has low levels of potassium on a regular basis, there is also the possibility of kidney failure.

Other normal medical problems and unfavorable side effects include:

- ❖ Weight gain
- ❖ Weakness and dizziness
- ❖ Stomach pain and bloating
- ❖ Rotting teeth and canker sores
- ❖ Swelling feet and hands
- ❖ Acid reflux and ulcers
- ❖ Recurrent sore throat and hoarseness
- ❖ Ruptured esophagus
- ❖ Broken blood vessels in the eyes
- ❖ Swollen cheeks and salivary glands
- ❖ Menstrual periods end
- ❖ Frequent constipation caused by laxatives

➢ The dangers of using Ipecac Syrup

If you use Ipecac Syrup to help you vomit after bingeing, be careful. Using this syrup on a regular basis can be deadly, as it builds up in the body over a period of time, leading to sudden cardiac arrest.

➢ Causes and risk factors of bulimia

There are many different factors that come into play when it comes to the cause of bulimia. Weight and the appearance of one's body image may be a major cause, but the inability to manage your emotions in a healthy manner also play a role. It's not surprising that people binge and purge when they're feeling angry, sad, tense, or anxious, because for them, eating can be an emotional release.

One thing we know for sure is that bulimia is a very complex emotional problem. Major causes and characteristics of bulimia are as follows:

- ❖ **Poor images of one's own body**

    The importance our society puts on being thin, and beautiful often cause young women in particular to be dissatisfied with their bodies, as they are bombarded with views of an unrealistic ideal of what they should look like.

- ❖ **Low self-esteem**

    Those at risk of bulimia include men and women who think of themselves as being useless, worthless, and unattractive. These people suffer from low self-esteem which is caused by depression, perfectionism, childhood abuse, and an unhealthy home atmosphere.

- ❖ **A history of trauma or abuse**

    Women in particular who have suffered from sexual abuse seem to have a greater occurrence of bulimia. Those who have parents that suffer with substance abuse or psychological disorder are also more likely to develop it.

- ❖ **Major life changes**

    Stressful changes or transitions in life such as children going into puberty, teens going away to college, or the breakup of a relationship often trigger bulimia. Bingeing and purging have been said to be a negative way of dealing with stress.

- ❖ **Professions and activities that require a certain appearance**

    People who are under pressure to look a certain way are exposed to the possibility of developing bulimia. The activities and professions that put them at risk include: ballet dancing, modeling, gymnastics, wrestling, running, and acting.

➢ **Getting help**

You understand how frightening bulimia can be if you have lived with it for any length of time, and knowing what you are doing to your body only increases the fear. But fear not, because it is possible for you to change. It doesn't matter how long you've suffered with bulimia it is possible to break the cycle of bingeing and purging, and create a healthier view of food and your body. It is natural to feel unsure about taking steps to give up bingeing and purging, and moving towards recovery can be a difficult process even though it's harming you. But remember, the very fact that you're thinking of getting help for this condition is a huge step forward.

➢ **Steps to recovery**

- ❖ **Admit you have a problem**

    The first step towards recovery is always admitting you have a problem and that your relationship with food is warped and out of control

- ❖ **Talk to someone about it**

    While it may be hard to talk to someone about something you've kept secret for such a long time, it's vital that you know you're not alone in this. So find someone you can trust and that you know will support you.

- ❖ **Avoid people, places, and activities that may cause you to want to binge or purge**

    Stay away from magazines that display fitness, and fashion, websites that mention weight loss, as well as friends that talk about weight loss. Take precautions when it comes to meal planning, cooking magazines and shows.

- ❖ **Seek help from professionals**

    When seeking advice, it is important to find someone who is trained to deal with eating disorders.

➢ **The importance of avoiding dieting**

The success of your treatment will be more likely to succeed if you eliminate dieting altogether. You will no longer feel overwhelmed with cravings and thinking about food, if you cease to put restrictions on the amount of calorie intake, and following rigid dietary rules. As you begin to eat normally again you can break the vicious cycle of bingeing, and purging and obtain a healthy, and attractive weight.

If you or someone you know has bulimia contact the National Eating Disorders Association at 1-800-931-2237 for referrals, advice and information.

➢ **Therapy and treatment**

It is critical to seek professional help early, so that you can deal with the root cause of your emotional problems that caused bulimia, and stop the vicious cycle of bingeing and purging. And it is equally important for you to see your treatment through to the end in order for it to be successful.

➢ **Therapy**

Therapy is a very important part of your recovery process, because it will help you sort out the issues you have such as, how you view your body, and low self-esteem, which lies at the heart of bulimia. Therapists can assist you in sorting out feelings of isolation and shame that developed as a result of your bingeing and purging. The best treatment for bulimia is cognitive-behavioral therapy, which focuses on the unhealthy eating habits of bulimia, as well as the impractical, and harmful thoughts that add to them. Therapy for bulimia includes:

❖ **Ending the cycle of bingeing and purging**

The first phase of treatment is directed towards ending the nasty cycle of bingeing and purging, and reinstating normal eating habits. The results that can be expected from therapy is as follows: learn how to watch your eating habits, stay away from circumstances that cause bingeing, deal with tension in ways that excludes food altogether, eat on a regular basis to decrease food cravings, and overcome your desire to purge.

❖ **Altering negative thoughts and patterns**

The second phase of treatment is directed towards recognizing and altering the unhealthy views when it comes to how much you weigh, dieting, and how your body is shaped. You also will take a look at different attitudes about eating, and reconsider the idea that some have, of self-worth being based on how much you weigh.

❖ **Solving emotional issues**

The final phase of treatment is directed towards targeting the various emotional problems that cause bulimia in first place. Therapy will may be centered on relationship problems, anxiety and depression, low self-esteem, and feeling isolated and lonely.

➢ **Helping someone with bulimia**

If you believe a friend or family member has bulimia, go to them and talk about your concerns. They might deny bingeing and a purging, but they may welcome the chance to talk about it. This shouldn't be overlooked because their physical and emotional health is at stake. It's hard to know that a loved on could be bingeing and purging, but you can't force them to change or do the recovery work for them. What you can do is offer compassion, encouragement, and support throughout the entire process.

> **Things you can do to help**
>   ❖ **Offer compassion and support**
>   ❖ **Avoid making insults, using scare tactics, sending them on guilt trips, and making patronizing comments**
>   ❖ **Set a good example for them**
>   ❖ **Accept that you are limited in what you can do**
>   ❖ **Take care of yourself**

Treatment providers
  ❖ **Eating Disorder Treatment Finder**
  ❖ **EDReferral.com**
  ❖ **National Eating Disorders Association**

Obsessive Compulsive Disorder (OCD)

It is normal that from time to time we will go back and make sure that the iron is unplugged, or that the front door is locked. But suffering from obsessive-compulsive disorder (OCD) where you have obsessive thoughts and compulsive behaviors, will literally cause interruptions in your life on a daily basis because it is so extreme. Just know that help is available, and with treatment and self-help techniques, it is possible to be set free from the barrage of undesired thoughts and illogical urges, and regain control of your life.

> **What is obsessive-compulsive disorder (OCD)?**

It is an anxiety disorder described by overwhelming, undesired thoughts and recurring behaviors that you feel forced to act upon. If you have OCD you most likely realize that your uncontrollable thoughts and obsessive behaviors are unreasonable, but even so, you feel helpless to stop. Just as a needle that gets stuck up on an old record, OCD causes the brain to become fixated on a certain thought. Some examples of OCD is checking 10 times to make sure you turned the light off down stairs, washing your hands repeatedly because they don't seem clean, or driving around for hours to make sure a particular sound you heard wasn't you running over an animal.

➤ Understanding OCD obsessions and urges

Obsessions are unintentional, seemingly overpowering thoughts, impressions, or urges that take place repeatedly in your mind. You don't desire to have these thoughts but you can't break free from them. And regrettably so they are often agitating and disruptive.

Compulsions are actions or customs you feel forced to act upon over and over again. These urges are normally acted out to try and make an urge to do something go away. An example of this is, if you're afraid of catching a disease, you might wear a mask and gloves every time you leave home. and with each occurrence the compulsive thoughts normally return greater. These behaviors usually end up triggering anxiety themselves as they become more insistent and consume more of your time.

The average person with OCD come under one of the following groups:

- ❖ **Washers**

    They're fearful of being polluted, and normally have urges to clean things or wash their hands

- ❖ **Checkers**

    They check things over and over that they connect with being injured or put in danger.

- ❖ **Doubters and sinners**

    They fear if they don't do everything perfect or in just the right way something bad might happen to them.

- ❖ **Counter and arrangers**

    For them everything has to be in a specific order or arrangement and must be equal in numbers for example. They might be delusional when it comes to certain numbers, colors, or arrangements.

- ❖ **Hoarders**

    They believe something bad may happen to them if they throw things away. They obsessively hold on to things that they don't need or use.

    Having obsessive thoughts and acting out compulsive behaviors don't necessarily mean you have OCD. With OCD these same thoughts and patterns cause an extreme amount of distress, consume much of your time, and disrupts your life and relationships on a daily basis.

➢ **Signs and symptoms of obsessive-compulsive disorder (OCD)**

On average people with OCD will have obsessions and compulsions as well, but some will experience one or the other.

➢ **Obsessive thoughts**

Normal compulsive thoughts in obsessive-compulsive disorder (OCD) include:

- ❖ Fear of being polluted by germs or polluting others
- ❖ Fear of hurting yourself or other people
- ❖ Having violent thoughts and imageries
- ❖ Focusing too much on moral ideas
- ❖ Having a fear of not having what they might need
- ❖ Oder and symmetry: everything must line up perfectly
- ❖ Superstitions: paying too much attention to be lucky or unlucky

➢ **Compulsive behaviors**

Normal obsessive behavioral patterns in OCD include:

- ❖ Repeatedly checking to see if family is safe
- ❖ Saying the same words over and over again to get rid of anxiety
- ❖ Repeatedly washing your hands or cleaning the house
- ❖ Putting things in just the right order

- ❖ Praying repeatedly or taking part in customs that are caused by religious fear
- ❖ Buying things just for the sake of having it, but never getting rid of
- ❖ Anything
- ❖ Repeatedly rechecking things like locks and appliances

> **Hoarding and other disorders**

Holding on to things that has little or know value is very normal for people with OCD even if it's not a severe condition, but those with symptoms of hoarding are generally suffering from things such as:

Depression, PTSD, phobia, skin picking, kleptomania. ADHD, tic disorders, or obsessive buying.

If you think you have you have OCD, let your doctor know about symptoms of hoarding, difficulty getting rid of junk, or fixating on losing things.

> **Obsessive-compulsive disorder symptoms and children**

OCD usually develop during adolescence or when children become young adults, sometimes the younger children may have symptoms that resemble OCD, however the symptoms of other disorders, like the following can also look like OCD, and they are: ADD, Autism, and Tourette's syndrome. For this reason, it is very important for them to have a thorough medical and psychological examination so that OCD can be ruled out and the proper diagnosis can be made.

> **Therapy as treatment for OCD**

Cognitive-behavioral therapy is the most effective treatment for OCD. Although medicine alone is rarely used for relieving OCD symptoms, there are times that antidepressants are used in conjunction with therapy.

> **Cognitive-behavioral therapy**

There are two different components that are involved in Cognitive-behavioral therapy for OCD and they are, exposure and response prevention, and cognitive therapy.

❖ **Exposure and response prevention**

This component involves being repeatedly exposed to your obsession, and refraining from the obsessive activities you would normally take part in, to reduce your anxiety. These activities include for example: Touching something you perceive to be dirty, and then not being able to wash your hands. As you sit endure the anxiety, the desire to wash your hands will eventually go away on its own. By doing this you find that it's not necessary to use this method to rid yourself of your anxiety, and that you do indeed have some control over your fixations and obsessive behavior.

❖ **Cognitive therapy**

This component involves focusing on disastrous thoughts, and the overwhelming sense of responsibility you feel. A huge part of this therapy is learning how to respond to your obsessive thoughts in ways that are both healthy, and effective, without giving in to your obsessive urges.

There are **four techniques** that can be used to overcome the symptoms of obsessive-compulsive behavior, and they are: **Relabeling, Reattributing, Refocusing and Revaluing.**

❖ **Relabeling**

Recognize that the obsessive thoughts, and desires that invade your mind are caused by OCD. An example is training yourself to say things like, I don't believe my hands are dirty, I don't really need to wash my hands, or what I'm sensing is only a compulsive urge to wash my hand.

❖ **Reattribute**

Realize that the power and invasiveness of the thoughts you have are the result of OCD, which is most likely linked to a biochemical imbalance in your brain. Tell yourself, this isn't me it's my OCD, in an effort to remind yourself that the thoughts, and urges you have from OCD doesn't mean anything, and that they are just false messages coming from your brain.

- ❖ **Refocus**

    Work around the thoughts you have as a result of OCD, by directing your attention to another area or subject for at least a few moments. Do something different. Tell yourself that what you're experiencing is simply a symptom of OCD, and that you need to take part in other activities.

- ❖ **Revalue**

    Don't take your thoughts that are associated with OCD at face value, because they are not important. Say things like, this is just that dumb obsession of mines, and it doesn't mean anything. It's all in my mind, and there is no reason for me to pay these thoughts any attention. Keep in mind, you may not be able to make the thought go away, but you don't have to entertain it either.

➢ **Family therapy**

Family therapy can be very helpful, since OCD often causes problems within the family structure. This type of therapy helps you gain an understanding of OCD and also helps to reduce family issues. In addition, it can both inspire family members, and teach them how to care for their loved one.

➢ **Group therapy**

As you interact with others who suffer from OCD, group therapy gives you the support and encouragement you need, and also reduces the feelings of isolation you may have.

➢ **Self-help Techniques**

If you are suffering from OCD there are many things you can do to help yourself, in addition to seeking therapy. The following are three self-help tips you can use to help you overcome OCD.

Tip #1

- **Challenging obsessive thoughts and compulsive behaviors**
  - **Refocus your attention**
  - When having compulsive thought and urges, you can attempt to refocus your attention on something else, for example:
  - Exercise daily, such as jogging or walking. Listen to music, read a book, surf the Internet, play video games, talk on the telephone, or take up a hobby such as knitting or other arts and crafts. It is important to do something you like doing for at least 15 minutes, so you can postpone your response to the compulsive thought or obsessive urge.
  - After you complete the act of postponing your thoughts and urges, reassess them. In most cases you will find that the desire isn't as intense as it once was. Repeat these actions, but this time try delaying for a longer period of time. The longer you are able to delay your desire, the more apt you are to change your response altogether.
  - **Write down your obsessive thoughts or concerns**

Be sure and keep paper and a pen handy, or even a laptop, smart phone, or a tablet. As you begin to have your obsessions, be sure to write down your thoughts.

- Continue to write your urges and record exactly what you're thinking even if you find yourself repeating the same phrases or urges over and over again.
- Writing everything down will help you discover just how repetitive your compulsions are
- As you write the same phrases hundreds of times, this will help your obsession lose its power.
- It is harder to write down your thoughts than it is to think them, so as you write them down they are more likely to disappear a lot quicker.

- ❖ **Anticipate having OCD urges**

    By expecting to have these urges you can help to relieve yourself of them. Make a mental note to tell yourself you have already completed the task you are obsessing with, and as you have the urge to obsess at a later time it will be easier to re-label it as an obsessive thought.

- ❖ **Create an OCD worry period**
- ❖ Instead of trying to hold back your obsessions, form a habit of postponing them for another time.
- ❖ Choose one or two "worry periods" everyday lasting 10 minutes each time, and make this time that you can dedicate to obsessing. Choose a time and a place, but make it early in the daytime so it won't affect your rest at night.
- ❖ During this time give your attention to negative thoughts and urges only. Don't attempt to correct them. Afterwards do some breathing exercises, release the urges and go back to your normal activities, but avoid obsessing for the rest of the day.
- ❖ As the thoughts come during the day don't forget to write them down and delay them to your worry period. Save it and go on with your day.
- ❖ Go over your list of worries, and reflect on the desires you recorded during the day. If they continue the concern you afterwards, allow yourself 10 minutes to obsess.
- ❖ **Create a CD of your obsessions**
- ❖ Think about a specific compulsion and record it.
- ❖ Recall the worry exactly as it comes into your mind.
- ❖ Playback the CD repeatedly for about 45 minutes every day, until listening to it no longer bothers you.
- ❖ As you confront yourself with your obsession, your anxiety will gradually wear off. Repeat the exercise using a different obsession each time.

Tip #2

> **Take care of yourself**

Having a healthy lifestyle will help keep your behavior, fears, and worries under control.

- ❖ **Practice relaxation methods**

    Although OCD isn't brought on by stress, any stressful situation can cause an onset of OCD, and make it worse.

- ❖ Do mind meditation, breathing techniques and other methods to help relieve your stress, and reduce your anxiety.

- ❖ Try relaxation techniques for 30 minutes each day, and eat healthy, starting with a good breakfast. Not eating regularly can lead to low blood sugar, and cause more anxiety.

- ❖ Eat a lot of carbohydrates like whole grain foods, also eat fruits, and vegetables. Complex carbohydrates will help alleviate high blood sugar, and boost serotonin levels.

- ❖ Exercise daily. Aerobics help relieve tension and stress, give you energy and release endorphins that help stimulate the brain.

- ❖ **Don't drink alcohol or smoke**

    Alcohol may reduce anxiety but will trigger it as it wears off, and nicotine is a powerful stimulant that causes high levels of anxiety and OCD symptoms.

- ❖ **Get proper amounts of sleep**

    A lack of sleep can cause anxiety, and proper amounts of rest will help balance you emotionally, and keep OCD symptoms under control.

Tip #3

> **Get support**

When you feel alone and powerless OCD can get worse, therefore it is vital for you to have a good support system. You will feel a lot less susceptible to injury when you are linked to other people and have someone you can talk to.

- ❖ **Stay linked up with family and friends**

    When you are alone OCD can consume your life, causing you to go into isolation, while aggravating your symptoms. Having a network of people who care is important, in terms of both support and treatment

- ❖ **Join a support group for OCD**

    It is important to know that you're not alone, and getting involved with support groups can not only act as a reminder of that, but you will also be able to interact with and learn from individuals who are suffering from OCD. You will also have the opportunity to share your own experiences, which could serve to help someone else.

➤ **Helping someone you love with OCD**

It is important for you to educate yourself about OCD if your loved one suffers from it. As you find information share it with them, and reassure them that help is available. Just knowing that it is treatable can give them a more positive outlook and motivate them to seek help.

➤ **Tips for helping a loved one with OCD**

Your negative reactions can hugely impact a loved one's OCD symptoms

- ❖ **Don't reprimand someone who is suffering from OCD**

    This is not a character flew, it is a disorder, and your pressuring them will make their behavior worse.

- ❖ **Be as kind and as patient as you can**

    Everyone recovers at a different pace. When they attempt to overcome their condition congratulate them, and direct your attention on the positive elements of what they're doing. This will encourage them to try harder.

❖ **Don't be a part of their rituals**

Being part of their ritual will only make things worse for them. Support them, not the disorder.

❖ **Make a deal not to let this condition overcome your family life**

Get together as a family and come up with a plan of how to deal with your loved one's condition. Try to keep things as normal as you possibly can, and find ways to keep the household stress to a minimum.

❖ **When talking be positive, direct and clear in what you say**

It is important to communicate about the OCD effectively, and without stressing out your loved one.

❖ **Find some humor in the situation**

Helping the loved one find some humor in their condition can be helpful in their ability to detach from it and recover. Remember, it is only humorous if they find it funny also.

Post-Traumatic Stress Disorder (PTSD)

When someone experiences a traumatic event, it is normal to feel a sense of fear, sadness, anxiety, and also to feel detached. But if the distress doesn't dissipate and you begin feeling as if you're stuck, and have continual feelings of danger along with painful memories, it could be that you have Post-Traumatic Stress Disorder or (PTSD). It may feel as if you will never get past what has happened or feel normal again, however if you seek treatment, get the support you need, and learn to develop new skills to help you deal with your condition, you can and will overcome PTSD and get on with your life.

➢ **What is post-traumatic stress disorder (PTSD)?**

Having a traumatic event happen in a person's life that threatens their safety, or makes them feel helpless can cause them to develop post-traumatic stress disorder. The average person links PTSD with soldiers that were scarred during battle, and the most common cause of PTSD in men is due to military combat, however it is a fact that any type of experience that causes trauma in someone's life can cause PTSD, and this is especially so if the event was unexpected, and something of which they had absolutely no control.

When it comes to PTSD it can have an effect on many people at one time, including those who personally experience the trauma, those who see it, and also those who help the person or persons involved pick up the pieces of their life afterwards. And this can also include emergency and law enforcement workers, and even the friends and family members of the one that was traumatized.

PTSD doesn't develop in everyone the same way. It usually appears very early on, as soon as a few hours or days following the event, but it can also take weeks, months, or years for it to show up.

➢ **Traumatic experiences that can cause post-traumatic stress disorder include:**

- **War**
- Natural disasters
- Rape
- Kidnapping
- Assault
- Car crash
- Plane crashes
- Terrorist attacks
- Sexual abuse
- Physical abuse
- Mental abuse
- Childhood neglect and abandonment
- Sudden death of someone you love

➢ What is the difference between post-traumatic stress disorder and a normal response to a trauma?

Traumatic events such those that cause PTSD are usually so catastrophic, and have such a great effect on people that they would cause emotional distress for anyone. Almost everyone that has a traumatic experience suffers from some of the symptoms of PTSD.

It is normal to feel unstable, fearful, detached, or numb when your sense of safety and trust has been destroyed. Other affects or normal reactions to such events can include having bad dreams, along with the inability to push what has happened out of your mind. These symptoms are short-lived for the average person, and may only last for a few days or maybe a few weeks, before they begin to disappear. If you are suffering from PSTD you'll find that you won't feel better as time goes by, but in fact you actually get worse.

When you become stuck that is when a normal response to trauma turns into PTSD

It is normal for your body and mind to be in shock after a traumatic event, and once you are able to process your emotions and make sense of what took place you will generally snap out of it. But if you develop PTSD the mental shock of everything remains, and your memory of what took place as well as your feelings about it becomes detached. And you will have to allow yourself to confront and deal with your memories of the event as well as your emotions.

➢ Signs and symptoms of PTSD

The thing about PTSD is that it doesn't always appear in the same scope of time, but it can come on you all of a sudden, gradually, and can also come and go over a period of time. Symptoms may also appear out of nowhere, but then there are times when something may happen that will remind you of the trauma, and this will trigger the symptoms. It could be a certain noise, an image, something that is said, or even a certain odor. Although it affects everyone differently, there are three key symptoms you can expect, which includes:

- ❖ Re-experiencing the traumatic event
- ❖ Avoiding what reminds you of the trauma
- ❖ Having an increase of anxiety and emotional stimulation

➢ **Re-experiencing the traumatic event**
- ❖ Having distressing memories invade your memory
- ❖ Having flashbacks or feeling as if it's taking place all over again
- ❖ Having nightmares of the event or something else scary
- ❖ Having anxiety attacks when you are reminded of what happened
- ❖ Having severe physical responses when reminded of the event, such as (heart pounding, heightened breathing, nausea, muscles tightens, or perspiring profusely)

- ❖ **Avoiding what reminds you of the trauma**
- ❖ Avoiding all areas, thoughts, sensations, and activities that remind you of the event
- ❖ Having memory lapses when it comes to important events surrounding the trauma
- ❖ Losing interest in the things you once loved to do and life in general
- ❖ Disconnecting yourself from loved ones and feeling emotionally numb
- ❖ Can't see yourself going anywhere in life, or not expecting to live long

➢ **Having an increase of anxiety and emotional stimulation**
- ❖ Insomnia
- ❖ Becoming touchy, with fits of rage
- ❖ Can't concentrate
- ❖ Always on the defense, or feelings of constant danger
- ❖ Easily scared and always tense

❖ **Other common symptoms**
❖ Angry
❖ Irritated
❖ Guilty
❖ Depressed
❖ Feeling hopeless
❖ Abusing drugs
❖ Feeling suicidal
❖ Unable to trust
❖ Feeling like no one wants you around
❖ Aches and pains

➢ **PTSD in children and adolescents**

In children, and those who are very young in particular, symptoms of PTSD can vary from those found in adults, and may include:

❖ Fearing being away from parents
❖ Not able to do the simplest things they've learned
❖ Insomnia and scary dreams that they can't remember when they awake
❖ Gloomy and obsessively acting out things that resemble the trauma
❖ Developing other fears and worries that are related to things unassociated to the trauma (fearing monsters, etc.)
❖ Acting out the event while playing, through telling stories, or through drawings
❖ Having pain in body for no good reason
❖ Displaying angry and irritation

➢ Causes and risk factors

No one can determine who will or will not develop PTSD after experiencing a trauma. But there are common risk factors that will increase your weaknesses, leaving you more open to injury, and a lot of the factors surround the nature of the event itself. If the event was very severe and posed a great threat to your life and well-being it is more likely to result in PTSD, and the more severe and lengthy threats generally put you at a greater risk of developing it. Cases such as rape, assault, and physical abuse or torture usually have a greater effect than acts of God, or incidents that were unintentional. Risks of developing PTSD are also greater depending on whether or not the event was unexpected, uncontrollable and inescapable.

➢ Other risks include:

- ❖ You had other traumatic experiences especially earlier in your life
- ❖ Family members had depression or PTSD
- ❖ Having suffered from depression, anxiety or other mental issues
- ❖ Having excessive stress levels daily
- ❖ No support after trauma
- ❖ Suffered from physical or sexual abuse
- ❖ Abused drugs
- ❖ Have no ability to cope with traumas

➢ Getting help

It is critical that you seek help immediately if you believe you or someone you know has PTSD, because the sooner you deal with it, the better your chances are of overcoming it. You must remember that PTSD isn't a sign of being weak, and that if you wish to overcome it you must be willing to face what happened and learn how to put it behind you. This is the only way you will be able to move on. It's common for you to want to bury painful memories and feelings and forget them, but this will only make it worse. It is impossible to get away from your emotions totally, you only wind up wearing yourself out, and once under stress they will emerge one way or another. Eventually you will ruin good relationships, putting your ability to function in danger, and your quality of life will suffer.

- **Why seek help?**
  - **The earlier the treatment the better**

    Dealing with your symptoms early will decrease the risk of PTSD getting worse

  - **PTSD can harm your family life**

    It can cause family members to back away from you as conflicts arise and get in the way of your relationships

  - **PTSD can cause other health problems**

    The condition can cause other health issues to get worse. It has been proven to be linked to heart problems

- **Treatment**

As you learn to cope with the experience of the trauma your symptoms will begin to subside. Treatment will help you to recall and process what you felt during the event so you can move past it, where you would otherwise try to avoid doing so altogether. Treatment not only helps you deal with the emotions you've locked up inside, but it will also help you regain control of your life, and decrease the great hold that the memory of the trauma has on you.

- **Treatment will help you:**
  - Take a look at your thoughts and emotions concerning the trauma
  - Work your way through feeling guilty, blaming yourself, and the inability to trust
  - Learn how to deal with and take control over memories that invade your thoughts
  - Confront and correct the problems you now have in your relationships

Mental Health Illnesses

- **Types of treatment**

  - **Trauma-focused cognitive –behavioral therapy**

    Involves carefully exposing yourself to thoughts, sensations, and circumstances little by little that reminds you of the traumatic event. It also helps you discover distressing thoughts about the event that are warped and unreasonable, so you can replace them with healthy ones.

  - **Family therapy**

    PTSD is especially damaging for you and your loved ones, and family therapy works to help you and your loved ones communicate better and work through your issues as you gain a better understanding of what you're dealing with

  - **Medication**

    Is used only to combat secondary symptoms such as depression. Antidepressants aren't usually given for PTSD because they do not treat the causes of it.

  - **EDMR or Eye Movement Desensitization and Reprocessing**

    Involves different elements of cognitive-behavioral therapy with eye movements or other methods of recurring, left-right encouragement, such as tapping the hands. This has been thought to work by relaxing the information processing system in the brain, which are disrupted when one experience great levels of stress.

- **Finding a therapist**

Always look for professionals that specialize in treating people suffering with PTSD and from trauma. Start with your primary care doctor. While it is important to find a therapy who has the right credentials and experience, you also want to find one that you will be comfortable with, and whom you feel you can trust. If you don't feel safe with them find another one, but don't give up on looking.

> **War Veterans with PTSD**

If you are a veteran and you have PTSD, there are centers that can help you get the counseling and other services you need.

> **Self-help treatment**

Recovering from PTSD is gradual and ongoing. Healing doesn't happen overnight and the trauma won't dissipate completely. Though it might make things hard for you at times, there are things you can do to deal with the symptoms that continue to linger, so you can decrease your depression and worry.

Tip #1

> **Seek support**

While you may be tempted to withdraw from others, and pull away from taking part in social activities, it is vital that you remain connected to those who care about you. Having people you can depend on when you need help is important for a successful recovery. Finding a support group for the same type of trauma is also important, and can be very helpful. You won't feel alone and isolated, and you can receive information that is vital for your recovery. Support groups are also available on line if you can't find one in the area where you live.

Tip #2

> **Avoid drugs and alcohol**

Although you might be tempted to self-medicate using drugs and alcohol, while struggling emotionally, it will only help you feel better temporarily but will make your PTSD worse. Using substances will make many of your symptoms worse such as depression, anger, and withdrawal. It disrupts your treatment and may cause additional problems at home.

Tip #3

> **Challenging the sense of helplessness you feel**

Since trauma already leaves you feeling helpless and powerless, it is important to gain a sense of power by strengthening your coping skills to get you through hard times. One of the easiest ways to regain a feeling of power to help others. Volunteering, giving blood, reaching out to assist someone in need, or giving to a favorite charity can give you a positive mindset, and help to challenge the feelings of helplessness resulting from PTSD.

Schizoid Personality Disorder

Schizoid personality disorder is one of a group of disorders called eccentric personality disorders, that cause people suffering from them to seem odd or peculiar. Those suffering from schizoid personality disorder have a tendency to be distant, disconnected, and uninterested in social circles or close relationships. These are people that are normally loners, who would much rather do things by themselves, almost never show strong emotion, and whose life is almost absent of any kind of pleasurable activities.

People suffering from SZPD seem unresponsive to the praise or critical comments that other's make. They normally appear very cold in nature, are almost never violent, and would rather not interact with people. Even though schizoid personality disorder and schizophrenia sound alike, and have some similar symptoms, these conditions are not the same. Most people suffering from SZPD are able to function pretty good, however they usually apply for jobs like night shift security officers, librarians or lab workers so they can be alone. Since people with this disorder rarely go for treatment, it's hard to accurately determine how wide spread it is. It affects more men than women, is more common in those who have relatives suffering from schizophrenia, and normally starts in early adulthood.

> ➢ **Signs and symptoms of Schizoid Personality Disorder**

Those who have SZPD often isolate themselves, and organize their lives very strategically to make sure they don't have to have any contact with other people. They never get married, remaining a resident of their parent's home throughout adulthood, are not very talkative, but daydream a lot and would rather deal in hypothetical situations to avoid becoming physically involved in any activities. In addition, they fantasize a lot in order to cope with their condition.

Additional symptoms of SZPD are as follows:

- ❖ They don't like or want to have intimate relationships with anyone at all, even family
- ❖ They choose activities and jobs that allows them to be alone
- ❖ They don't like to partake in activities, including sex
- ❖ Their only friends are immediate family members
- ❖ They can't function well around others
- ❖ They could care less about receiving praise and criticism
- ❖ They are very distant and cold
- ❖ They daydream a lot, living in a world of fantasies

➢ **Causes of Schizoid Personality Disorder**

There isn't much known about the cause of SZPD, but it is said that genetics and the environment one lives in plays a major role. It is believed by some mental health professionals that growing up in a household where the environment is full of sadness or misery, absent of love and where no form of emotions is displayed, is a contributing factor for developing Schizoid Personality Disorder. It is also suspected that one of the major causes is genetics, based on the fact that those having family members that suffer from schizophrenia have been known to develop schizoid personality disorder.

➢ **Risk factors linked to Schizoid Personality Disorder**

It is a great likelihood that those who were isolated throughout their childhood, subjected to living with parents who were withdrawn, uncaring and disconnected from other people, and then encouraged to be the same would develop SZPD traits.

➢ **Diagnosing Schizoid personality disorder**

No one has pin pointed a specific set of laboratory tests for SZPD, and it's not until after a thorough clinical review has been conducted, that a diagnosis can be made. During the interview questions will be asked concerning one's symptoms, mental well-being and also their medical, psychiatric, and social history. In addition, a physical examination should be done in order to help rule out other conditions they may possibly have.

A person must meet four of the following criteria in order to be diagnosed with SZPD:

- ❖ Doesn't enjoy or want to be involved in close relationships, even if it's family
- ❖ Whenever choosing activities or jobs they are always away from other people
- ❖ Almost never has a desire to be sexually active with another person
- ❖ Rarely takes pleasure in any activities, and almost never shows emotions
- ❖ Isn't close to anyone other than family
- ❖ Doesn't seem to care about receiving praise or criticism
- ❖ Is very aloof and disconnected

In addition, the person must not have symptoms exclusively while having a bout of schizophrenia, mood disorders while displaying psychotic characteristics, a different psychotic disorder or a persistent developmental disorder such as autism. It isn't befitting to make a diagnosis if the symptoms are caused by a medical condition that is directly related to their psychological issues.

Because schizoid personality disorder mimics autism and Asperger's syndrome, this further complicates the diagnosis.

➤ Treating SZPD

People suffering from SZPD can't see that they have a problem, and therefore don't feel like they need to undergo treatment, and because of this they usually won't show up for their sessions. Their family and friends usually have more of a concern for their isolation than they do. It is vital that you don't make the assumption that persons with SZPD are just withdrawn, shy, or merely insecure. People with these traits can possibly be diagnosed with Avoidant Personality Disorder, which isn't necessarily the case. Those suffering from SZPD can have problems communicating with the therapist while in treatment, and may respond in a wishy-washy, disconnected manner. But when they are shown respect for their personal space they can respond to their treatment in a very positive manner.

People with SZPD are normally treated with psychotherapy such as: Psychodynamic therapy and group therapy. Cognitive-behavioral therapy can also be quite effective in helping them change their thinking and behavioral patterns, since personality disorders lead to inaccurate thought patterns. Even though persons with SZPD don't have the ability to increase their desire to become socially involved with others, they can become proficient enough to connect with, talk to and get a long with others. And though they may not desire to create intimate relationships they often have a desire to connect with other people, and be more successful at being comfortable with others. In this respect role-playing can be quite useful.

When taking part in group therapy, little by little patients can create self-disclosure, feel the interest of other suffering with SZPD, and practice interacting while receiving an immediate response from others. No specific drug is used for SZPD, but anti-depressants, anti-psychotics, and anti-anxiety medications are normally used in conjunction with therapy, to relieve symptoms of depression and anxiety that are associated with their condition. Medications are best used in conjunction with therapy and should not be used by themselves when treating SZPD and other personality disorders.

Schizophrenia

Schizophrenia is a disorder that challenges you, making it hard to determine whether something is fact or fiction, think clearly, cope with your emotions, connect with others, and operate normally. But still there is hope because you can successfully manage schizophrenia.

There are three step to successfully managing schizophrenia and they are:

- ❖ Identifying the signs and symptoms
- ❖ Seeking help without delay
- ❖ Sticking with the treatment

Getting the correct treatment and support can help someone suffering from schizophrenia lead a happy, fulfilling life.

➢ What is schizophrenia?

Schizophrenia is a brain disorder that gives people an altered since of reality, often with a significant loss of what is really real, and also affects the way they act, think, and view the world. This disorder causes those suffering from it to hear things that aren't there, say things that are very confusing, accuse people of trying to harm them, or feel as if they are being watched all of the time. Because the line between what is factual and what is fiction is so blurred, schizophrenia makes it hard and even scary to navigate their daily activities in life. In turn those with schizophrenia will often pull away from others or do things out of fear and confusion.

Many times, cases of schizophrenia tend to show up in people that are in their late teens or early adulthood, but it could appear for the first in those who are also middle aged or older. Even though it's rare, schizophrenia affects young children and adolescents, but the symptoms are somewhat different. It normally has a greater affect on men than it does women, and affects those that develop it early in life more than others.

Even though it is a chronic disorder, help is available for schizophrenia. People can function independently and live a satisfying life, if they receive the right support, medicine, and therapy. The best chance for managing schizophrenia is having it diagnosed and treated immediately. Many treatments are available, and chances of recovery are good, if you or your loved one gets help as soon as the signs, and symptoms of this disorder are spotted.

➢ Common misunderstandings about schizophrenia

There are different myths concerning schizophrenia and they include the following:

Myth #1 Schizophrenia is the same as split or multiple personalities

Fact

Multiple personality disorder is very different from schizophrenia and a lot less common, and those suffering from schizophrenia don't have split personalities, instead they are separated from reality.

Myth #2 Schizophrenia is a rare disorder

Fact

Schizophrenia isn't a rare condition; the odds of someone developing it throughout their lifetime are 1 out of 100.

Myth #3 Those suffering from schizophrenia are dangerous

Fact

Even though the unrealistic thoughts and illusions of schizophrenia can cause one to behave violently, many that are diagnosed with it aren't aggressive, or a threat to others.

Myth #4 Those with schizophrenia cannot be helped

Fact

Even though treatment for schizophrenia may be a lengthy process, there is hope for those diagnosed with it, to have a joyful life and function properly both within their communities and their family.

> **Early warning signs**

Although schizophrenia normally shows up at a moments notice, giving no warning, for most people, the onset of it is slow, and the warning signs sneaks up on you, causing your ability to function in a normal mental capacity to decline, long before you ever have the first dangerous occurrence. Many times those who have a loved one with schizophrenia will report that, they suspected something was wrong with them, but they didn't know what it was.

In the early phases of schizophrenia those who have it will often appear to be strange, uninterested in things they once loved, and will also lack emotions. They will withdraw from people, stop keeping up their appearance, say things that are strange, and act as if life is insignificant. They may turn away from hobbies and activities they once took part in, and their job performance, and grades declines.

The most widespread early warning signs include:
- Withdrawing from social activities
- Becoming suspicious
- Bad personal hygiene
- Unexcited, lifeless stare
- Unable to cry or show happiness
- Crying or laughing at inconvenient moments
- Depression
- Insomnia or excessive sleeping
- Making strange statements
- No ability to concentrate
- Overacting to criticism
- Babbling; saying things that make no sense

➢ **Signs and symptoms**

When dealing with symptoms of schizophrenia, there are five characteristics you can look for and they are:

Delusions, hallucinations, disorganized speech, disorganized behavior, and the so-called negative symptoms

When it comes to the patterns and severity of the symptoms, they show up very differently from person to person, may change over time, and then there are those who will have some of the symptoms, but not all of them.

- **Delusions**

This is an idea that a person holds on to in spite of the fact that it is very clear that it's not true. Delusions are very normal for those with schizophrenia, involving unreasonable views or ideas, while affecting over 90% of those who have it.

The following are a list of common schizophrenic delusions:

- **Delusions of persecution**

    Believing that people are out to get them, while creating crazy ideas in their head such as UFO's are landing in their back yard waiting to beam them up.

- **Delusions of reference**

    An impartial place or event is believed to mean something special, such as someone on TV, or the radio is sending subliminal messages just for them

- **Delusions of Grandeur**

    Believing that they have supernatural powers, and can jump from buildings without dying, or that they're someone very important like Jesus or the President.

- **Delusions of control**

    Believing some outside source is controlling their thoughts or actions, like aliens.

    The devil is making them kill people.

- **Hallucinations**

Sounds that seem real, but are only so in their mind. Even though hallucinations can generally involve any one of the five senses, auditory, and visual hallucinations are usually common in people with schizophrenia. These hallucinations may not mean anything to someone else, but they mean a lot to them, and usually sound like someone they know. The voices are usually life threatening, abusive, or Ill-mannered, and normally get worse when they're alone.

➢ Disorganized Speech

One of the characteristics of schizophrenia is fragmented thinking, which will hinder the ability to focus and maintain a train of thought, and can be detected when one speaks. Those with schizophrenia often respond to questions with answers that are totally unrelated to what's being asked, or begin a sentence with a specific subject in mind, and then veer off on a topic that's completely different.

Some of the normal signs of disorganized speech are:

❖ Loose or unattached Associations

This is where a person jumps from one subject to another at a rapid pace, and as they speak their thoughts are confused, having no connection with one another.

❖ Neologisms

Creating words and expressions that only mean something to them.

❖ Perseveration

Making the same statement over and over again.

❖ Clang

Using rhymes that make no sense and are absolutely meaningless (e.g. The man can ban at the pan and all I can see is Dan).

➢ Disorganized behavior

When you set goals for yourself schizophrenia will interfere with them, hindering your ability to care for yourself, work a job, and have a conversation with or do things with other people.

Disorganized behavior is viewed as:

- ❖ A decrease in one's complete ability to function on a daily basis
- ❖ Having random responses
- ❖ Acting strange and making no sense in what you do
- ❖ Being unable to keep urges under control and have no shame

➢ **So-called negative symptoms (absence of normal behavior)**

With schizophrenia, the term so-called negative symptoms signify the normal behaviors that have disappeared, and are no longer evident in people that are healthy.

Some normal negative symptoms of schizophrenia are:

❖ **Inability to express emotions**

No facial expressions or a blank stare, no excitement in the voice, and no eye contact

❖ **No enthusiasm**

Unable to motivate or care for oneself

❖ **Disinterest in what's going on the world**

Have no idea what's going on in one's environment, and keeping to oneself

❖ **Difficulty communicating with others**

Giving strange responses to question asked, and difficulty holding a conversation

➢ **Causes of Schizophrenia**

While it may appear that schizophrenia is developed when both genetic and environmental issues are present, it is not fully known what causes it.

➢ **Genetic causes**

Schizophrenia is in general a hereditary disorder, and those who have relatives that have it such as a parent or a sibling, have a 10% chance of developing it as opposed to the usual 1% chance worldwide. It is important to note that this disorder isn't determined by genetics, but merely influenced by them, and though it runs in the family nearly 60% of those who have it have no family members with it. In addition to that, many that are susceptible to develop the disorder don't get it, and this shows that biology doesn't determine your destiny.

➢ Environmental causes

Studies that have been done on twins, and those adopted shows that genetics causes one to be at risk of developing schizophrenia, and then the environment that people find themselves subjected to such as stress and late stages of pregnancy works together with this vulnerability to trigger schizophrenia. When Cortisol, a hormone that is produced by the body increases, because of high levels of stress, this also causes schizophrenia to develop.

According to research there are several environmental factors that induce stress, and may be involved in schizophrenia and they are:

- ❖ Being exposed to a virus-related infection while pregnant
- ❖ Having your oxygen levels decrease as a result of prolonged labor during birth or premature birth
- ❖ Being exposed to a virus as an infant
- ❖ Losing a parent or being separated from one as a child
- ❖ Being abused physically or sexually abused as a child

➢ Abnormal structure

Abnormal brain structure, just as abnormal brain chemistry may also play a role in developing schizophrenia. Some schizophrenics have been known to have, enlarged brain ventricles, indicating that there is a shortage in the volume of brain tissue. It has also been said that the activity in the frontal lobe, which is the area of the brain responsible for reasoning, planning, and making decisions is abnormally low. Research has also shown that brain abnormalities in the temporal lobes, the hippocampus, and the amygdala are linked to developing schizophrenia, but regardless of this evidence concerning brain abnormalities, it is very questionable whether this disorder is the result of any single issue in any single area of the brain.

❖ Effects of schizophrenia

It is important to note that, whenever the signs and symptoms of schizophrenia go undetected, and ignored or are improperly treated, this can be very dangerous and also devastating, not only for the person with the disorder but also for the people around them.

Here are some possible effects:

❖ **Relationship issues**

Because people with schizophrenia often withdraw, isolate themselves from other people, and deal with suspicions, relationships will generally suffer.

❖ **An interruption of normal daily activities**

The schizophrenia delusions, hallucinations, and disorganized thoughts that normally keep a person from performing ordinary things like bathing, eating, or running errands can cause substantial interruptions to everyday functions, both because of the difficulty they have with socializing, and because daily tasks simply become tough, if not impossible to do.

❖ **Alcohol and drug abuse**

Those with schizophrenia often develop issues with substance abuse, which are normally used to try and self-medicate or relieve symptoms. If they turn to smoking it could be a complicated situation because nicotine can interfere with how effective the medicine prescribed will be.

❖ **Higher risk of suicide**

Schizophrenics are at a great risk of attempting suicide, and are are especially prone to commit suicide during psychotic occurrences, bouts of depression, and in the first 6 months of treatment, and if there is any talk of suicide, any threats, or any comments about suicide it should be taken very seriously.

Diagnosing schizophrenia

Diagnosing This disorder is diagnosed based on a **full psychiatric evaluation, medical history, physical examination, and lab tests.**

Mental Health Illnesses

- ❖ **Psychiatric evaluation**

    You will be asked a series of questions about you or your loved one's psychiatric history.

- ❖ **Medical exam**

    You will be asked about your family health history, and you will receive a complete physical to check for medical problems causing the condition.

- ❖ **Lab tests**

    Blood and urine tests are taken to rule out other medical causes and symptoms, although there are no lab tests that can diagnose schizophrenia. You may undergo tests such as, CAT scan or MRI to look for brain abnormalities connected with the disorder.

➢ **Criteria used to diagnose schizophrenia**

If you have at least 30 of the following symptoms you could have

Schizophrenia:

- ❖ Hallucinations
- ❖ Delusions
- ❖ Disorganized speech
- ❖ Disorganized behavior
- ❖ Negative symptoms (isolation, uninterested, lack of communication)
- ❖ **Important problems functioning**

    At school or work

- ❖ **Reoccurring signs**

    6 months with active signs and symptoms

- ❖ **No diagnosis can be made by tests**

    There are no tests that can diagnose Schizophrenia

The medical and psychological conditions the doctor must rule out before diagnosing schizophrenia include:

- ❖ **Other psychological disorders**
- ❖ **Substance abuse**
- ❖ **Medical conditions**
- ❖ **Mood disorders**
- ❖ **PTSD Post-traumatic stress disorder**
- ❖ **An accident**
- ❖ **Violent assault**

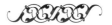

CHAPTER 11

Emotional and Psychological Trauma

➢ **How emotional and psychological trauma works**

Not all potentially traumatic events lead to lasting emotional and psychological damage. Some people rebound quickly from the most tragic experiences, but things that appear to be less upsetting on the surface devastate some. There are a number of risk factors that can make people susceptible to emotional and psychological trauma. For example, if someone is presently under heavy stress and have already experienced a number of different losses, they will most likely be traumatized by a single stressful experience. People who have already experienced trauma and especially those who have experienced these events in their childhood, are more likely to be effected by a new situation.

People react in different ways when it comes to trauma, and can experience wide variety of emotional reactions. When experiencing trauma no one can really be prepared for certain events, and no one can really say how they would react or how someone else should react. So one should not judge their self on how they react nor should they judge anyone else on how they react, after all, these are normal reactions to abnormal experiences that they now have to try and mentally digest, and also make the necessary adjustments.

Some of the typical reactions one can expect from emotional and psychological distress are:

- ❖ Shock and disbelief
- ❖ Confusion, and difficulty concentrating

- ❖ Anxiety and fear
- ❖ Feeling sad, hopeless, or worthless
- ❖ Guilt, shame, or self-blame
- ❖ Anger, irritability, and mood swings
- ❖ Withdrawing from others
- ❖ Feeling numb, empty, and disconnected

Typically, these symptoms can last from a few days to a few months, but may continue to resurface over time, and can be triggered by certain dates, words, events, or situations that remind you of your painful experience. Recovering from a traumatic event takes time, and everyone heals at a different pace. If you notice that a significant amount of time has passed, and you're still struggling with your symptoms without any relief, this is evidence that it is time to seek professional help.

Some of the symptoms that you can look for to determine whether or not to seek help are:

- ❖ Having trouble functioning at home or work
- ❖ Suffering from fear, anxiety, or depression
- ❖ Unable to form close relationships
- ❖ Having terrifying memories, nightmare

When you experience traumatic events as a child you can have a severe and long-lasting effect. Children are very trusting and fragile, when violated their sense of security can be greatly affected and they will begin to see the world as a very frightening and dangerous place. When the trauma is not resolved this fear and helplessness will carry over into their adulthood, and set the stage for them to be introduced to more emotional trauma.

Childhood distress can be a result of things such as:

- ❖ Unstable environments
- ❖ Divorce

- ❖ Sexual, physical and verbal abuse
- ❖ Domestic violence
- ❖ Neglect
- ❖ Abandonment
- ❖ Bullying

Following are some of the traumatic events that many will experience throughout their life.

Abandonment

Abandonment is not only a common problem for children, but it's also an issue for adults and the elderly. It refers to the absence of emotional support, and physical absence as well. Just about everyone deals with the fear of having to live life all alone. How abandonment affects someone may vary from person to person, and having the support of people who love you is very helpful when coping with it. When abandonment starts affecting one's life on a deep level, it is usually noticeable because of its ability to control their thoughts and actions. The symptoms abandonment issues normally begin to appear as the person starts to feel deprived of love and support.

> **Children and abandonment**

When a child suffers the loss of one or both of their parents, he or she feels abandoned, and this condition is known as abandonment child syndrome. Medically speaking abandonment is a form of psychological disorder. Whenever a child has been given up for adoption, the feeling of bereavement causes them to feel abandoned. Physical abandonment is felt when there are parents who are too busy, and never find time for their children.

Children can begin feeling emotionally abandoned when experiencing problems in the family such as a lack of bonding, and having to see their parents fight all of the time, or being deprived of love for any reason can trigger these feelings.

- **Visual symptoms**
  - ❖ **Sickness**

    The child is more likely to become sick very often because of the mental stress of being abandoned. They will normally withdraw from general activities due to their mental state, and being unable to cope with rejection.

  - ❖ **Lack of concentration**

    Because of the chaos in the home it will be difficult for the child to focus on their schoolwork, and activities and they probably won't feel like doing anything else, resulting in poor performance and low grades.

  - ❖ **Negativity**

    When a child is dealing with rejection, they can very easily develop a negative attitude, and may become frustrated and easily angry over petty issues.

  - ❖ **Disorders**

    Children dealing with abandonment may begin to eat poorly due to depression, and may also suffer from insomnia.

  - ❖ **Behavior**

    Abandoned children often retreat to things such as: crying, daydreaming, wetting the bed, sucking their thumb, becoming possessive of a certain toy, blanket or pillow, having temper tantrums, and if one parent leaves they will often fear losing the other parent also. They may also begin to fear the darkness.

  - ❖ **How to help**

    The earlier feelings of abandonment are detected the easier it is to help a person recover, preferably at childhood. When you realize that your child feels abandoned, it is important to gain his or her trust, so start bonding with them to let them know that they are not alone, that you will always be there for them, and that they will not have to face the world alone.

It is important for you to encourage your child to participate in social activities, and help direct them in their schoolwork, by doing so this will help to improve their self-confidence. But if their behavior doesn't change seek professional help.

- **Adults and abandonment**

People are normally able to recognize their own faults and weaknesses, as they grow older. The fear of being rejected or abandoned for the same reason is likely to overcome them. In addition, if the person was abandoned as a child, the sense of fear that they feel can become deeply rooted, and develop a strong hold on them. Experiencing the great pain and disappointment, that comes from losing someone close or being rejected by a loved one, could very well lead to abandonment issues over a period of time. Abandonment in adults can result in them developing serious mental, emotional, and physical problems.

- **Visible symptoms**
  - **Worthlessness**

    Considering the fact that the one being abandoned, isn't counted as being worthy of their loved one's love, time, and attention, they will begin to question their own significance and value. If there is an unfaithful spouse or a friend that turned their back on them, this could also trigger feelings of worthlessness, causing them to oversimplify their actions, and begin blaming their self.

  - **Guilt**

    The person will begin to believe the abandonment came as a result of something they have done. It could also cause them to try and figure out what they have done wrong, and feel guilty for something that isn't their fault.

  - **Insecurity**

    This is where the person grows up feeling insecure, and that it is necessary to always cling to other people. Because of this fear they may hold too tightly to people in an effort to hold on to them, but in the long run could cause problems in their relationships

❖ **Withdrawal**

Feeling insecure could make one feel second-rate, causing them to remove their self from participating in social activities, and the fear of rejection will hinder their ability to mingle with others. In almost every case, the fear of abandonment will cause a person to feel as if their partner would leave them, so they will break off the relationship first.

❖ **Bad habits**

An adult struggling with abandonment may consider drinking alcohol and doing drugs, as a way of coping with their fears and issues. In believing no one else cares about them, they won't care much about themselves.

❖ **Excessive Reassurance**

Because of abandonment, it can be hard for a person to trust again, and believe they can find someone that will love them, because of this they are always seeking to be reassured.

❖ **Being self-complacent**

Those suffering from abandonment can become very complacent (e.g. not caring what others think about their actions and their appearance, enjoying partaking in repulsive household duties and sexual activities, which their significant other may not like.

❖ **Low self-esteem**

Someone who suffers with abandonment issues will usually have low self-esteem, which leads to being insecure, feeling as if they can't do anything, and also depression.

➢ **How to help**

Becoming attached to people isn't healthy, so it would be best to avoid doing so. When you detach yourself from someone it doesn't mean you no longer care, you're just maintaining a safe distance so that you don't become reliant on others. Because focusing on the future and keeping your mind on the life you are presently living is important, it would be a good idea to find things to keep you busy, this will help you keep your mind off of your negative past experiences. Exercising, getting into sports, starting a new hobby, or doing things with your friends are good examples of things to do. Setting, and finishing goals that will make you feel good about yourself is also helpful. If all of this fails, and nothing else seems to help, you may want to seek a professional.

> **Elderly people and abandonment**

When people reach a certain age, they begin to feel worthless, and as their body starts giving out on them, and they begin to lose their mental faculties and their strength, they will often feel fruitless. This will cause them to sink into depression. It is at this point that they need to be loved, accepted, and supported by their family. If they become isolated and are rejected they can begin to feel abandoned, and rightly so. There are many reasons why elderly people may be abandoned. For example; many children are ungrateful, uncaring, and selfish, feeling that they are just too busy, and never finding time for them.

> **Visible symptoms**

❖ **Depression**

As an elderly person, the thought of living a life of loneliness can be very fearful, and when faced with the challenge of being alone it can cause them to go into depression.

They are also faced with symptoms such as low self-esteem, worthlessness, loss of appetite, sluggishness, withdrawal, and insomnia.

> **How to help**

Being abandoned can be overwhelming for the elderly, however to get over their feelings of depression they can take part in different activities such as, knitting, stitching, and other crafts or hobbies. This will help take their mind off of being alone. They can also try making new friends to spend time with, and going for walks to relax their mind.

Caregiver Burnout Stress

If you feel like the caregiving situation you're in has taken control of your life, and you're in over your head, you can become very overwhelmed to say the least. If the stress of caring for a loved one is left unchecked, it can and will take a toll on your health, your relationships, and your state of mind and will eventually lead to a burnout. When a person is burned out, it's tough for them to do anything, let alone look after someone else. For this reason, making time to rest, relax, and recharge is no longer a luxury, but has now become a necessity.

> **Understanding Caregiver Stress and Burnout**

Although caring for a loved one can be very rewarding, it can also involve many stress factors that include:

- ❖ A change in the family dynamic
- ❖ Household disruption
- ❖ Financial pressure
- ❖ An added workload

When considering this one does not have to wonder why people who are caregivers are among those that are most prone to burnout.

Caregiving is a challenge that is usually chronic and long-term, simply because it is something that one may face for years and even decades, and the stress of it can be particularly damaging. When dealing with a situation like this, if there is no hope that your family member will get any better, it can be very disheartening, and unless you have the help and support you need, the stress of it can leave you very vulnerable to a vast amount of physical and emotional issues, that can range anywhere from heart disease to depression.

As a caregiver, if your health is affected your ability to provide care will also be affected, therefore it not only hurts you but also the one you're caring for. The point I'm making is that caregivers need care also. If you're going to stay healthy, you must manage your health. This is just as important as making sure your family member goes to their doctor's appointment and takes his or her medication on time.

➢ **Signs and symptoms of caregiver stress and burnout**

The first step to coping with the problem is learning to recognize the signs of caregiver stress and burnout.

➢ **Common signs and symptoms of caregiver stress**
- ❖ Problems thinking and concentrating
- ❖ Increased resentment
- ❖ Drinking, smoking or eating more
- ❖ Neglecting responsibilities
- ❖ Cutting back on leisure activities
- ❖ Anxiety
- ❖ Depression
- ❖ Irritability
- ❖ Feeling tired and run down
- ❖ Overreacting to minor nuisances
- ❖ New or worsening health problems

➢ **Common signs and symptoms of caregiver burnout**
- ❖ Having a lot less energy than you once had
- ❖ It seems like your resistance is down and you catch every cold or flu that's going around
- ❖ You're tired all of the time, even after sleeping or taking a break
- ❖ You don't do things for yourself, either because you're too busy or you don't care anymore
- ❖ Everything you do is scheduled around caregiving, but it gives you little satisfaction

- ❖ You find it hard to relax, even when help is available
- ❖ You have little or no patience
- ❖ You begin feeling helpless and hopeless

When you are burned out caregiving is no longer healthy for you or the loved one you're caring for. Therefore, it is very vital for you to be aware of the warning signs of caregiver burnout, so that you can recognize the problem and take the proper precaution right away.

It's okay to ask for help

It is important not to try and take on the responsibility of caring for someone by yourself, because it will result in a burnout. Instead, try enlisting the assistance of others to help out with the cooking and errands, and make sure to take breaks as often as possible.

Tip #1

➢ **Getting help**

- ❖ **Speak up**

    Your family and friends won't automatically know what you are in need of or what you feel, so don't expect them to. Come forward and tell them what's going on with you and your loved one that's receiving the care. If you feel there are some things that can be done differently to help your situation, voice your opinion no matter how they may respond. It is important to start dialoguing about it to get the support you need.

- ❖ **Share the responsibility**

    Contact family members and get them involved in the care of your loved one as much as possible. It doesn't matter how far away they live, there is something that even they can do. Set up a schedule and dole out different responsibilities for everyone according to what they're able to do.

❖ **Have someone check up on you regularly**

Have someone call you as often as you think you need them to, that will be able to call family, and friends and give them a status update and also help you coordinate the help you need.

❖ **Don't turn down help when it's offered**

If someone offers to help you don't turn it down. Make them feel good about wanting to support you, by accepting the help they offer. Make a list of things you need help with and heave it ready, so as people call you can easily tell them what you need without having to think about it.

❖ **It's okay to relinquish some control**

People will be more willing to help if you make them feel like you're working together, rather than micromanaging everything that's done, giving them orders and insisting that everything is done your way. It's okay to ask for suggestions. This will make them feel more like a partner.

Tip #2

➢ **Give yourself a break**

Time for rest and relaxation may seem like a luxury that you don't have as a busy caregiver, but it's something that you not only owe to yourself, you also owe it to the person you're caring for, to make this part of your schedule as well. If you would allow yourself time on a daily basis, to rest and do some things that you enjoy doing, it will make your job as a caregiver less stressful, and you will be a better caregiver because of it.

You can actually be busy and not be productive. Therefore, if you continue on with your responsibilities as a caregiver without taking time off to de-stress and recharge, you actually end up getting less work done in the long run. If you take a break and allow yourself to get the proper amount of rest, afterwards you'll find yourself feeling more energetic, focused and able to quickly make up for the time you took to rest.

❖ **Set aside at least 30 a day for yourself**

You owe it to yourself to do things you enjoy, whether it's exercising, reading, sewing, walking, working in the garden or watching television.

❖ **Pamper yourself**

It doesn't have to be anything lavish, small luxuries can be very big in relieving stress and picking up your spirits. You can do things such as taking a candle lite bath, get a massage or get your nails and hair done, whatever makes you feel good.

❖ **Find ways to make yourself laugh**

It is said that laughter is good for the soul. It is also good medicine for stress. Try indulging in something that will make you laugh, by watching a funny movie, reading a funny book, going to see a stand up comedian or see a play based on comedy. It also helps to try and find humor in everyday matters if you can or call a friend that has the ability to make you laugh.

❖ **Plan an outing**

Ask family and friends to give you a break so you can have some time away from home.

❖ **Go and talk to friends and tell them what you're feeling**

Sharing your feelings or venting can be very therapeutic. If you don't have anyone to sit with your loved one, invite a friend over for a visit, and make dinner or coffee. It is vital for you to interact with other people. Though you may feel you're being a burden to your friends, you will find that most of them will be delighted at the thought, that you would trust them enough to tell them what you're dealing with, and this could even serve to strengthen your relationship with them.

Tip #3

> ### Practice accepting the situation

When you find yourself confronted with the burden of caring for a sick or disabled loved one, in an effort to make sense of it you may find yourself asking "why?" but when it comes to things you can't change, it is fruitless to spend a lot of time dwelling on it, because it won't make you feel any better, and especially when it's something about which you can find no clear cut answers. What you should do instead, is try to avoid falling into the emotional trap of feeling sorry for yourself or having pity parties. And focus your attention on accepting where you are in life, while seeking for ways that you can grow from it.

❖ **Focus on what you can control**

None of us can change things we have no control of no matter how much we worry or focus on it, so instead of becoming stressed out over what you can't control, focus on the things you can change and on that which is positive.

❖ **Seek to find the silver lining**

Focus on how being a caregiver has changed you for the better, or how you've become closer to or mended the relationship with your loved one. Think about the pros of caregiving such as, how you have been able to show your love for that person by giving back to them the same love they have given to you over the years.

❖ **Share what you're feeling**

Although you can't change your situation, it can be quite therapeutic just to talk about. Find someone you can confide in and share what you're going through.

❖ **Try to avoid having tunnel vision**

Instead of allowing caregiving to consume you and take control of your life, you can help make the situation easier to deal with by doing things that can give your life purpose and meaning. Some examples of what you can do are: starting a new career, going back to school, and finding new interests such as a relationship or new hobbies. Go to church, and develop a relationship with God and allow him to give you strength and new direction.

Tip #4

➤ **Take care of your health**

Just like a car, if you take care of your body it will remain in good condition, and generally won't break down on you, but if you don't take care of it you can begin having multiple problems with it. It is important that you don't do anything that will add to the already stressful situation you're dealing with, by allowing your health to go bad.

❖ **Don't neglect to keep your doctors appointments**

If you're not healthy you will be of no use to your loved one or yourself. While it may be easy to overlook your own well-being when you're consumed with caring for your loved one, be careful not to. You matter too, so be sure you go to all of your check-ups and other medical appointments.

❖ **Exercise regularly**

When you are stressed out and worn down it is hard to get motivated to exercise, but this is exactly what you need and you will feel great afterwards. Exercise helps relieve stress and enhance your mood. Try to workout for at least 30 minutes a day. You will find yourself feeling more energetic and less fatigue.

❖ **Meditation**

Meditation or daily relaxation can help relieve stress, and there are many different techniques you can use such as: deep breathing, muscle relaxation and even listening to calming music. For some people sitting by the water can be relaxing and you can also try reading bible passages and meditating on the word of God.

- ❖ **Eat right**

    It is important to nourish your body by making sure you eat the right foods. The following is a list of some healthy foods you can eat. Vegetables, whole grains, beans, lean protein, healthy fats such as nuts and olive oil. These foods will help to give your body energy that will last.

- ❖ **Get the proper amount of sleep**

    Most people don't know it but cutting back on your sleep is unhealthy, and when you do so it can be counterproductive, especially if your goal is to get more work done. Though the average person gets less, 8 hours is what is needed for the body to be at its best, and anything less will cause your mood to change, your energy level to be lowered, your productivity to suffer and also hinder your ability to handle stress.

Tip #5

- ➢ **Join a support group**

As a caregiver, support is a must, and finding a support group will be one of the most important things you can do for yourself. This is a great way to share the problems you encounter as a caregiver, and interact with people who go through the same things that you do each day. For those who have no way of getting away from home there are many internet groups available also. These groups give you the opportunity, to not only talk about your problems, but also listen to others, learn from them and even be a help to those listening to you. During these group sessions you will come to know that you are not alone in what you're dealing with, and that there are others who are dealing with the exact situation as yours, and who's knowledge can be very valuable to you.

Child Abuse and Neglect

Although physical abuse may be more visible than the scars of emotional abuse and neglect, these types of abuse leaves deep scars that last a long time. Children who are abused have a greater chance of healing, and breaking the vicious cycle of becoming an abuser, if they are treated early. And one can make a big difference in a child's life, by learning the common signs of abuse, and what they can do to help.

➢ **Understanding child abuse and neglect**

Child abuse consists of more than just bruises, and fractured bones, and while people may think that it is so obvious because of the scars that physical abuse leaves, it isn't. If you ignore the needs of a child, put them in danger by leaving them unsupervised, or make them feel as if they are worthless or dumb, it is considered child abuse. It doesn't matter what type of abuse a child is subjected to, all abuse will still cause serious emotional harm.

➢ **Myths and facts**

Myth #1 Violence is the only type of abuse

Fact

Abuse doesn't just consist of being physically assaulted it also includes neglect, and emotional abuse, which can cause just as much damage. And people aren't as likely to step in, because it is so subtle.

Myth #2 Children are only abused by bad people

Fact

It is easy for people to make comments such as, only bad parents abuse their children, because abuse isn't always what it seems to be in the sense that, not everyone that harms their children are doing it intentionally. There are many people who were also abused as children, and because of this they are parenting the only way they know how. While there are those who suffer from mental health illnesses or substance abuse issues.

Myth #3 There is no child abuse among good families

Fact

Child abuse isn't prejudice. It happens in all families whether rich or poor, in all neighborhoods whether good or bad, and touches all races, economic levels, and cultures. In fact, those who seem to have it all together tend to live a totally different kind of life behind closed doors.

Myth #4 Most children are abused by strangers

Fact

Although strangers abuse many children, it is usually those who are closest to them, such as family and close friends that abuse the most.

Myth #5 Children who were abused will always become abusers themselves.

Fact

Even though abused children are more apt to grow up, and unconsciously repeat what they were subjected to by becoming an abuser, there are many parents that survived child abuse, who are not only great parents, but are also strong advocates for abused children, and will go to great lengths to protect their own children from being abused.

> **Effects of abuse and neglect**

Although many child abuse scars are physical, and all types of child abuse and neglect may leave scars that last a long time, the kind of scarring that effects people all throughout their life, and damages a child's sense of self, their ability to conduct a healthy relationship with other people, and to function properly at home, work or school is emotional scarring.

Some of those effects include:

❖ **Having a lack of trust and relationship issues**

When the person responsible for their care abuses a child, it will wound the most basic relationship that they can have. They will no longer trust you, the person that is supposed to protect them with their physical safety. Without being able to trust those who are supposed to love them, it will be almost impossible for them to learn how to trust other people, or to know who is really trustworthy at all. Because they now have a fear of being abused or controlled, this will make it very hard for them to conduct a relationship. And because they have no idea what a good relationship is, this can lead to a string of unhealthy ones.

- ❖ **Feeling worthless or damaged**

    Being told over and over again as a child that you are ignorant, or no good, makes it quite difficult to get past these feelings, and they can easily become a reality for you. As an adult you probably won't excel in the area of education, or you may even settle for a low paying job, because you don't feel worthy of a better one or that you're capable of exceling to a higher level in life. Those struggling with feelings of being damaged or ashamed are usually people who have been sexually abuse.

- ❖ **Trouble managing one's emotions**

    As a result of being abused, the emotions of a child may become suppressed, and begin surfacing in unexpected ways, and in addition to this they're not able to safely to express their emotions. Adults that were abused as a child will often have problems with anxiety attacks that they're unable to explain, depression, or bouts of anger. Because of this they will resort to alcohol or drugs to get rid of the pain.

➢ **Types of child abuse**

Although there are many types of child abuse, the essential component that bonds them all together is the emotional affects they have on a child. Children feel safest in environments where there is predictability and things don't change from week to week, a strong foundation, clear-cut boundaries, and where they know that their parents will look out for them and keep them safe. Parents that are abusive, live in a world that is unpredictable, scary, and without rules and their children can never predict how they will react. It doesn't matter if the abuse is a slap across the face, a nasty comment, cold silence or wondering if they will have food on the table at dinner time, at the end of the day all of it leaves the child feeling unsafe, uncared for, and alone.

> **Emotional child abuse**

Emotional abuse has the ability to greatly damage a child's mental health or their social growth or expansion, resulting in emotional scars throughout their entire life.

Some examples of emotional abuse are:

- Constant putting down, embarrassing, and degrading a child.
- Calling them nasty names and comparing them to others in a negative manner.
- Telling a child they are no good, that they don't mean anything, they're bad, or that giving birth to them was a mistake.
- Yelling all of the time, making threats, or bullying them
- Not paying the child any attention or rejecting them as a way of punishing them.
- Not showing the child and love or affection; no hugs or kisses.
- Putting the child in dangerous situations where they are in the midst of abusive situations

> **Child Neglect**

Child neglect is a type of abuse that is quite common, where a parent provides inadequate care for their children, when it comes to food, clothing, hygiene, or supervision, and is not always noticeable. Parents who neglect their children may be struggling with illnesses such as depression, anxiety, alcohol abuse, or drug addiction. Older children will become accustomed to their neglect, putting a smile on their face, acting as if nothing is wrong and taking on the role and responsibility of a parent.

> **Physical abuse**

Physical abuse includes harming a child physically or injuring them, and while it is sometimes deliberate, this isn't always the case. The abuse may also be the result of severe discipline, such as using a belt, or physical punishment that is inappropriate for the child's age or physical condition. Many parents, and caregivers that abuse their children claim that what they use is simply a method of discipline, to help the child learn how to behave, but there is a very big difference between punishing a child physically as a way to discipline them, and physically abusing them. The whole reason for disciplining children is to help them learn right from wrong, not to cause them to live their life in fear.

> **Physical abuse vs. Discipline**

When it comes to physical abuse, rather than physical discipline, some of the components you will see are:

- ❖ **Unpredictability**

    There are no clear boundaries or rules when it comes to physical abuse. The child is always walking on eggshells, never knowing what will set the parent off, or what will trigger a physical assault.

- ❖ **Striking out in anger**

    Parents who abuse their children normally act out of anger, and the urge to affirm their control, rather than the drive to teach the child in a loving manner. As the parent grows more and more angry, the abuse becomes worse.

- ❖ **The use of fear to control behavior**

    Physically abusive parents might believe they need to instill fear in their children to get them to behave therefore, they will use physical abuse to keep the child in order. But in essence, the child isn't learning how to behave, instead they are learning how to avoid being hit.

- ❖ **Child sexual abuse**

    Child sexual abuse is a very complex method of abuse because of its many layers of guilt and embarrassment. It is vital to understand that one does not have to have bodily contact in order to be sexually abused. If a child is subjected to a situation surrounding sex or sexual material it is still considered sexual abuse even if there is no bodily contact.

It is a frightening thing to hear stories about sexual predators on the news, but it's even more fearful to know that someone they know, such as a close family, or someone else they should be able to trust normally sexually abuses children. And contrary to popular belief, girls aren't the only ones who are sexually abused, it happens to boys also. As a matter of fact, when boys are sexually abused it isn't always reported, because of the disgrace and humiliation they stand to face.

> **The issues of shame and guilt when it comes to child sexual abuse**

While the physical damage of child sexual abuse is powerful, the emotional trauma of it is just as damaging and also far-reaching. Children who are sexually abused may feel that they are at fault for what happened to them, and are tortured with feelings of guilt and shame. They might also feel that they are somehow responsible for the one that abused them. This can cause them to have issues with sex, such as extreme acts of promiscuity or being unable to engage in intimate relations, and can also lead to self-hatred. It is very difficult for children to report sexual abuse because of the shame they feel. They could also be concerned that their family might bee torn apart, that no one will believe them, or that someone might be angry with them. Now that you're aware of how difficult it is for a child to report this type of abuse, understand that it is uncommon for them to falsify such accusations, so if a child tells you they've been sexually assaulted, please take them seriously.

> **Warning signs**

Child abuse isn't always noticeable, but the earlier it is identified the better chance the child will have of receiving proper treatment and recovering. The possibility of identifying the problem early on and helping both the child, and the abuser get the help they need, will become greater, if you are able to understand the common warning signs of child sexual abuse. Be careful not to jump to conclusions, because the fact that you see a warning sigh doesn't necessarily mean a child is being abused, so it is vital that you look deeper into the situation, and try to identify whether or not there is a pattern of abusive behavior, and warning signs.

- **Warning signs of emotional abuse**
  - Extremely withdrawn, scared, or worried about doing the wrong thing.
  - Displays excessive behavior such as, being excessively demanding, passive, or aggressive.
  - Emotionally detached from the parent or caregiver.
  - Acts too adult or too much like a baby (rocking, sucking their thumb, or throwing tantrums)

- **Warning signs of physical abuse**
  - Always being injured, bruises they can't explain, swelling, or cuts.
  - Always on edge
  - Patterned marks on the body (such as injuries from a hand or belt)
  - Doesn't want to be touched, jumps when sudden moves are made, or doesn't want to go home.
  - Always wears clothing such as long sleeves when it's hot, to cover up injuries.

- **Warning signs of neglect**
  - Clothes are dirty, raggedy or improper for the weather.
  - Bad bodily odors, not bathed, dirty or matted hair.
  - Illnesses and injuries that go untreated.
  - Left home alone a lot, subjected to unsafe environments or situations.
  - Misses or comes late for school on a consistent basis.

- **Warning signs of sexual abuse**
  - Difficulty walking or sitting.
  - Takes an interest in or has knowledge of sexual acts that they shouldn't know about or acting seductive.
  - Try very hard to avoid being around a certain person for no good reason.

- ❖ Doesn't want anyone to see their body or take part in activities that require body contact.
- ❖ They get pregnant or a sexually transmitted disease at 14 or younger
- ❖ Often runs away from home

➢ **Risk factors for abuse and neglect**

Though child abuse and neglect takes place all types of families, even in the families that seem happy, there are certain situations in which children are at a much greater risk such as:

- ❖ **Domestic violence**

    For children, witnessing something such as domestic abuse is not only torturous, but also emotionally abusive. This type of situation does extensive damage to a child, even if the parent is successful in keeping them from being physically abused. The best way to protect your child if you are in an abusive relationship is to get out of it.

- ❖ **Alcohol and drug abuse**

    It is very hard for a child that is living with and alcoholic or drug addict, because they could very easily be abused and neglected. Parents who are constantly drunk or high lack the ability to properly care of their children, make the right decisions for them, and manage inclinations that can cause danger. Those who abuse substances may also physically abuse their children.

- ❖ **Untreated mental illnesses**

    Parents who suffers from mental illnesses such as anxiety, or bipolar are often unable to take care of themselves, and their children. If a parent is mentally ill, under the influence of drugs, or have been traumatized, without even understanding why, they will become detached, withdrawn, and also quick to become angry with their child.

❖ **Lack parenting skills**

There are some parents such as those who are teens, who simply never grasped the necessary skills for good parenting, and are therefore naïve when it comes to the needs of a child or a baby. Or if the parent of a child was also a victim of abuse as a child, their experience in caring for their children will most likely be based on how they were raised. In these types of cases, the parent can improve their skills of parenting, by tapping into sources such as parenting classes, therapy, and caregiver support groups.

❖ **Stress and lack of support**

Parenting can be quite difficult, especially if you are dealing with relationship issues, financial hardships, or raising a child without the help of family and friends. If your child is disabled, has special needs, or difficulty with their behavior, it is vital that you get the proper assistance, so that you will be able to give your child the emotional and physical support they need.

➢ **Recognizing your own abusive behavior**

If you feel angry, need help and resources, and live in the U.S., but don't know how to get it, you can call 1800-4-A-child to find out what sources are available in your community, to help you overcome the cycle of abuse in your life. For helplines that are available in other countries you can visit: **Chiworld.org**

Raising children can be a challenge, and may cause people with the mildest temper to become angry and frustrated, and if you grew up in a home where the normal way of living was to scream and shout, this is probably the only way you know to raise your children. One of the most difficult situations for a child is being raised in an abusive environment, and the biggest step you can take towards getting help is first identifying that you have a problem.

Depending upon the kind of environment you grew up in, that would determine what would be the norm for you, for example: if in your family you and your siblings were slapped, or shoved for no apparent reason, your mother was always so drunk that she couldn't cook dinner, your parents constantly called you dumb, or stupid, or you watched your father beat your mother on a regular basis, these experiences became a normal way of life for you.

Once we become adults we then have the ability to take a step back, and take a closer look at what is considered to be normal, or abusive. Take a look at the types of abuse and warning signs above, and ask yourself if any of them look familiar to you now, or from when you grew up. Below is a list of warning signs that let you know if you might be journeying into the area of abuse.

You have crossed the line of abuse if:

- ❖ **You can't control your anger**

  You may begin with one smack on the buttocks, but find yourself hitting your child multiple times and each time it gets harder. You find yourself shaking him or her and then throwing them on the floor. Or you begin screaming, and then find yourself getting louder and unable to stop.

- ❖ **You have become emotionally detached from your child**

  You have become emotionally overcome by your situation, and don't want to deal with your child at all. More and more each day all you want is for them to be quiet, and leave you alone.

- ❖ **It as become impossible to meet your child's daily needs**

  Everyone struggles with the daily job of getting their children dressed, feeding them, and getting them off to school or to after school activities, but if you find that you can no longer achieve these goals, this is a sign that you may have a problem.

- ❖ **Other people have shown their concern**

  Denial is a common reaction, and while it may be easy to recoil or get offended when people express their concern, you must carefully consider what is being said to you, and whether or not the people who are voicing their concerns are someone you trust and respect.

➢ **Breaking the cycle of abuse**

If you were abused as a child, giving birth to children of your own may trigger powerful memories and feelings that you may have bottled-up. It can take place when you have a child, or later on in life as you recall specific abuse that you endured. These feelings may cause you to become shocked and overcome by your anger, and you may feel as if you can't control it, but it is possible for you to learn different ways to cope with your emotions, and break your old patterns.

It is important to remember that the most important person in your child's life is you. They are worth the effort that is necessary to make a change, and you don't have to do this alone.

➢ **Tips to help you change your reactions**

❖ **Learn what is and is not age appropriate**

Having an accurate perception of what you should realistically expect of your child can help you avoid becoming frustrated, and angry at what is simply normal child-like behavior. For example, it isn't natural for a newborn baby to sleep all night without waking up, and small children don't have the ability to sit still, and be quite for a long period of time.

❖ **Developing new parenting skills**

Although it is important for you to learn how to manage your emotions, you must also have a plan in place for what you will do instead. You can begin by turning to sources such as parenting classes, books, or seminars to learn proper methods of discipline.

❖ **Take care of yourself**

When you don't get proper amounts of rest you can begin to feel overwhelmed, and will be more apt to give in to your anger. A lack of rest only adds to your irritability.

- ❖ **Seek professional help**

    It can be quite hard to break the cycle of abuse if the patterns are deeply rooted. If you find that you can't stop abusing no matter how hard you try, this is a sign that it's time to get help whether it is therapy, a parenting class, or other methods of help.

- ❖ **Learn to control your emotions**

    Realizing that you have emotional issues is the first step to gaining control of them. If for example you had to curb your emotions as a child, you may now have a problem holding them back.

➢ **How to help an abused or neglected child**

If a child tells you they're being abused, it's normal to feel somewhat overwhelmed and perplexed, and it can be hard to accept or talk about child abuse. This may be your chance to make a huge difference in the life of a child that's being abused, especially if you take the necessary actions to end the abuse early on. Reassuring the child and giving them unconditional support as you talk to them is the best thing you can give them. Since it is difficult for a child to talk about abuse, in the first place, your job is to reassure them and do whatever you can to help.

➢ **Tips for talking to a child who's been abused**

- ❖ Avoid denial and remain calm
- ❖ Don't interrogate the child
- ❖ Reassure them that they didn't do anything wrong
- ❖ The child's safety always comes first

➢ **Making an anonymous report**

It is vital to get the help a child needs, if you feel they are being abused. Making a child abuse report may seem very formal, and a lot of people don't like to get involved in other family's private affairs, so they may be hesitant to do so.

The following are some of the myths people have about reporting child abuse:

- ❖ **I don't want to intrude in someone else's family affairs**

    The damage that child abuse does to a child is far-reaching, and can not only affect future relationships, and the child's self-esteem, but if the cycle continues other children could also be at risk.

- ❖ **I might break up someone's home**

    Since the child protective service's priority is keeping the child in their home, making a report doesn't necessarily mean they will automatically be removed. It will only result in removal if the child is in clear danger

- ❖ **They will know that I was the one who called**

    When reporting child abuse it is anonymous, and you are not obligated to give your name when reporting, therefore no one can find out it was you.

- ❖ **What I have to say won't make a difference**

    If you feel something is wrong, better safe than sorry. You may not be able to see the entire picture, but the fact is that there may be other's who have noticed things also, and seeing a pattern can help identify abuse that would otherwise go un-noticed.

➢ **When reporting abuse**

Because reporting abuse can cause a lot of emotions and uncertainty to surface, you will probably ask yourself if what you're doing is right, or if anyone will listen to you.

The following are tips for effectively communicating when the situation is tough:

- ❖ Try to be as precise as you can
- ❖ No that you may never find out what the outcome will be
- ❖ Continue to report other incidences if you notice any

➢ Reporting abuse that took place in your home or child custody

When you witness abuse at home or think abuse is taking place in a child custody situation, it can be challenging to say the least. You may fear what will happen to you or your children if you say something, or you might be worried the abuser might cover their tracks or even blame you, and cause you to wind up losing your children.

➢ How to report an abuse in the home or in child custody cases

- ❖ Stay calm
- ❖ If it's an emergency dial 911
- ❖ Write everything down that you've seen
- ❖ Get your child an evaluation
- ❖ Start an investigation
- ❖ Go to CPS
- ❖ Seek an attorney
- ❖ Contact JUSTICE FOR CHILDREN at 1800-733-0059 if you have a problem completing steps 3-6. M-F 8-5 CST

Child Abuse Hotlines:

- ❖ US or Canada: 1-800-422-4453
- ❖ UK: 0800 1111
- ❖ Australia: 1800 688 009
- ❖ New Zealand: 0800-543-754
- ❖ Other international helplines: ChiWorld.org

Help for child sexual abuse:

- ❖ 1-888-PREVENT (1-888-773-8368) Stop It Now
- ❖ 1-800-656-HOPE Rape, Abuse & Incest National Network (RAINN)
- ❖ Or visit ChiWorld.org for a list of other international child helplines.

Divorce/ Breakup

> ### How to Cope with a Breakup or Divorce

Moving on from a marriage or love relationship is never easy no matter what happened. Ending a relationship can affect every area of your life, stir up many different emotions that are difficult to deal with, and also cause you much pain. As painful as it may be this experience can actually help to strengthen and educate you, and there are many things you can do to help you get past this phase of your life and move forward.

> ### A time of healing

Whether the relationship has gone sour or not, loss is not easy to accept. Many breakups are difficult because of the heart felt commitment, and all of the time, planning and effort that is spent when two people merge their lives together. Most relationship starts out on a very positive note, with both parties full of enthusiasm and hope for a bright future together. The loss of a relationship can be much like experiencing a death, causing one to go through a period of mourning, which brings with it much pain and disappointment.

Many people lose their identity while in a relationship, and a breakup can cause your life to spiral downward. It will cause great hardship for you, making it difficult to function in other relationships, at work, at home, totally disrupting your daily activities. Breakups also have the ability to bring you to a place of uncertainty, causing you to question yourself about many things. You can begin to wonder how would you function without your partner, whether or not you would ever find love again, how would you handle being alone. These thoughts can be torturous.

Though it may be a difficult time, it is important to keep in mind that healing might be slow, but it's possible, and that life does go on and you can and will survive with or without them.

➢ **Learning to Cope with separation and divorce**

❖ **Understand that it's OK to feel different**

During a breakup there are certain feelings that are normal. Some are feelings of sadness, weariness, frustration, anger, and even confusion. There are times when anxiety may set in, as you think about your future and what it may hold for you, but over a period of time you will experience them lesser, and lesser. It is okay to admit that you're afraid of moving forward. This is generally because you have no idea what lies ahead.

❖ **It's okay to take a break**

At times like this it is normal to have a lower level of energy or enthusiasm, causing you to operate at a slower pace, and slack off from some of the things you're accustomed to doing. You are only human, and it will take a while for you to regain your strength and momentum, so don't stress yourself out by feeling like you must function as if everything is okay because you don't. if necessary take some time to be by yourself and sort things out.

❖ **Don't go through this by yourself**

It's not healthy to endure this process alone. It is necessary to vent and share your feelings and pain with those who love you, so that you can be successful in surviving this breakup. When you suppress your feelings you can set yourself up for stress elevation, which can lead to emotional illness, and affect your ability to focus, disrupt other areas of your life such as work and even affect your overall health. There are also support groups that are available to you if you need them, where you can interact with others who have had a similar experience.

➢ **It's okay to grieve the loss of your relationship**

Grieving is not only a normal part of the process when a love relationship is dissolved, but it also includes a number of losses such as:

- ❖ Loss of companionship
- ❖ Loss of support. For example, financial and moral support, and social and emotional support
- ❖ Loss of hopes and dreams that you thought would become a reality, and the time and energy put into the relationship

Though it might be a scary time for you it's okay to allow yourself time to grieve, because it's necessary for your healing process in the sense that it enables you to move on from past relationships, and as painful as it might be you can rest assure that it won't last forever.

➢ **Tips for grieving**

❖ **Don't fight your feelings**

The grieving process consists of ups and downs coupled with a gamut of different emotions, such as fear anger and confusion. It is essential to your healing process for you to not only recognize these emotions but to also acknowledge them. While they may be painful if you suppress them it can and will be harmful to your emotional state, and will also cause you to grieve longer than necessary.

❖ **Express how you feel**

Not everyone is able to talk about how talk to others about what they're feeling, but it is an essential part of the grieving process, and will help you heal when you learn that others are aware of your pain and you're not alone in what you're dealing with. Another way to release your feelings is to journal.

❖ **Remember that your goal is to move on and not get stuck in your grief**

While it is essential for you to express what you're feeling, don't get stuck in an emotional state by dwelling on negative feelings and over-emphasizing your situation, and robbing yourself of the positive energy needed to move forward.

❖ **Remind yourself that your life has not ended**

When you make a commitment, by buying into a person and into a relationship with them, together you create a hope for the future, and it's not easy to let go of. Keep in mind that just as you created hopes and dreams with that person the world has not come to an end, and as long as you're still alive you can create others.

❖ **Know the difference between a normal reaction to a breakup and**

don't allow yourself to become delusional, where you can no longer tell the difference between a normal and abnormal reaction to a breakup.

If you're not careful your grief can easily cause you to plummet into a place of depression.

➢ **Taking care of yourself after a divorce or relationship breakup**

When going through a divorce it can be a very stressful, and emotional ordeal and also life changing. Because of the mental health issues that are connected to emotional stress, it is important to take good care of yourself during this period. Taking care of yourself will consist of reduce your sources of stress, both mental and physical.

➢ **Self-care tips**

❖ **Make time each day**

Do things to encourage yourself, and that will make you feel better both physically and mentally.

Examples: walking, music, relaxation,

❖ **Pay attention to what you need**

If you feel something is good and best for you, don't allow others to put you on a guilt trip. It's okay to say no to others at the risk of doing what is best for yourself.

- ❖ **Stick to a routine**

  Routine displays normalcy in an individual, and getting back to yours helps to eliminate the chaos, stress, and uncertainty that disrupts your life as a result of a divorce.

- ❖ **Take a time out**

  Making major decisions when you are emotionally stressed can lead to bad decisions, so take the time to rest until you feel confident, that your decisions will be made based on what you know rather than what you feel.

- ❖ **Avoid using alcohol, drugs, or food to cope**

  The use of alcohol, drugs, and food to cope with the pain of your divorce can become a crutch and a danger to your health over time. It is so important to seek out other ways that are healthier.

- ❖ **Explore new interests**

  Rather than looking at a divorce as the end of your life, take a second look and begin to view it as the beginning of something new. It is healthy to begin exploring new love interests, and new activities in an effort t regain your life.

- ❖ **Making healthy choices:** Eat well, sleep well, and exercise

➢ **Important lessons learned from a divorce or breakup**

In times of emotional crisis, there is an opportunity to grow and learn. Just because you are feeling emptiness in your life right now, doesn't mean that nothing is happening or that things will never change. Consider this period a time-out, a time for sowing the seeds for new growth. You can emerge from this experience knowing yourself better and feeling stronger.

Gaining an understanding of why something happened, and how what you did contributed, coupled with acknowledging the part you played, and then learning from your mistakes will be key to moving forward with your new life.

Some questions to ask yourself

- ❖ Have you bothered to take a step back and look at the entire picture?
- ❖ Ask yourself if you tend to repeat the same mistakes or continually choose the wrong person in relationships?
- ❖ Take a look inside yourself and ask have you done all that you could to protect the relationship?
- ❖ Do you tend to accept other people the way they are, or do you try and make them what you want them to be?
- ❖ Do your feelings, and emotions control you or do you control them?

➢ **Children & Divorce**

It's never easy when a divorce or the breakup of a significant relationship takes place, and the situation can be especially difficult when a child is involved. Children need both stability and support, but it's hard to give them what they need when your emotions are all over the place, you're sorting out the final details of a divorce and possibly dealing with an ex who is resolved to give you a hard time.

It is possible to be successful in assuring your children that they are loved, and helping them remain strong throughout this difficult time, but it won't be possible unless you take care of yourself. Children are resilient, but can also be very fragile, however with your help they will be able to come through this process unscathed.

Helping Children Cope with Separation and Divorce

No matter what age they are, divorce can affect children in the same stressful way that it affects you, not only causing them to experience feelings of sadness and confusion, but also pain which is associated with the anger and realization that their parents will be separating for good. By covering and nurturing them you can help make their grieving process as painless as possible. In order for this to happen it is important that they see you maintaining a positive attitude, and that you assure them that you will provide a place of stability.

As a parent, you won't have all of the answers, nor will you always know exactly how to help your child cope with divorce. However, though you may feel as if you're walking in unfamiliar territory, you can be successful navigating through it.

There are a variety of ways you can assist your children in adjusting to separation or divorce. As You listen to them, continue to be patient, and give them the reassurance they need, the amount of tension they feel can be limited, while making it easier for them to learn how to cope with this and other new situations. You can do this by structuring a consistent routine, and maintaining a positive stress free relationship with your ex. Although you can't totally eliminate the pain and difficulty they will face in this time of transition, as you make their well-being your priority it will help to minimize the amount of damage they receive.

➤ **What a child need and want from both parents**
- ❖ Stay involved, it makes them feel truly loved and important
- ❖ Maintain contact, and communicate regularly
- ❖ Ask questions, it shows that you're interested
- ❖ Don't fight with one another, when you do your child thinks it's their fault and feels guilty.
- ❖ Be able to agree on matters that concern your child.
- ❖ Don't make your child feel guilty about spending time with the other parent, as this makes them feel like they need to choose between you.
- ❖ Keep communication with your ex open, and don't send messages through the child.
- ❖ Don't say anything bad about your ex in front of your child. They may feel like you want them to take sides with you against their other parent.
- ❖ The child needs and wants both parents to play a role in raising them, so please work together.

➤ **What to tell your kids**

When telling your child about the divorce make sure you prepare ahead of time what you will say, and anticipate what they might ask you so that you will be prepared to answer their question, and help them cope with the news.

> **What to say and how to say it**

Don't try to protect them by making up a story, and make it as easy as possible for them to understand

- ❖ **Tell the truth**
- ❖ Be honest with them, but make your explanation short and simple so they don't get confused, and assure them that their relationship with both parents will remain intact.
- ❖ **Say "I love you often"**

  It is crucial that you reassure your child that your love for them will never change.

- ❖ **Address changes**

  Gently break the news that you will no longer be living together under in the same house, but let them know they will still spend plenty of time with each parent.

- ❖ **Avoid blaming**

  Be honest but don't be critical of your ex when giving an explanation of the divorce to your child.

- ❖ **Present a united front**

  Come together as a unit for the sake of giving the same explanation.

- ❖ **Plan your conversations**

  Tell your child about the new living arrangements before they take place, and if possible do it together.

- ❖ **Show restraint**

  Be fair and respectful of the other parent when giving an explanation for the separation.

➢ **How much information to give**

It is not necessary to tell them everything at once, it can be too much to handle.

❖ **Be age-aware** How much information you give should be based upon their age.

❖ **Share logistical information**

It's important to tell them about any changes in living arrangements, school, and daily activities, but keep it minimal.

➢ **Helping children cope by listening and reassuring them**

Children need to be able to have an outlet to express their emotions, and they need you to help them do so. This can be done by committing to listen to what they have to say, and not become defensive. It is your job to help rid them of their fears by giving them the reassurance they need, clearing up any misunderstandings they may have, letting them know that they had nothing to do with your marriage coming to an end and that you love them no matter what.

➢ **Children need to express their feelings**

Divorce can make children feel like they've lost everything; the life they knew, and even their parents. But you can be there for them by being the support system they need; helping them cope with the grieving process, and adjust to this new set of circumstances they're facing.

❖ **Listen**

Children may have feelings of sadness, loss and frustration, and it is important to encourage your child to share their feelings, when they do make sure you listen.

❖ **Help them find words for their feelings**

Children tend to have a problem articulating what they feel, so it is important to take notice of your child's moods and encourage them to speak out.

❖ **Allow them to be honest**

Children are sometimes hesitant to express their true feelings for fear of hurting you. It's important to let them know that it's okay to say what's on their mind. This will enable them work through what they're feeling without too much difficulty.

❖ **Acknowledge what they're feeling**

Although you can't fix your child's problems or turn their sadness into happiness, it will make a difference to them if you acknowledge what they feel. Instead of dismissing what they say listen, because in doing so you help them build a relationship of trust with you.

➢ **Clearing up all misunderstandings**

Many kids believe that they had something to do with the divorce, recalling times they argued with their parents, received poor grades, or got in trouble. You can help your kids let go of this misconception.

❖ **Setting the record straight**

Make sure they understand why you got a divorce. This can be a great help for them.

❖ **Show patience**

Kids are not mature enough to fully comprehend certain circumstances. One day they seem to grasp everything and the next day they're not so sure. It is important for you to be patient with them, and eventually it will all sink in.

❖ **Reassure your child**

It is vital for your child's well-being, that you constantly reassure them that they had nothing to do with your divorce, and that you love them very much.

- **Give reassurance and love**

By reassuring your child of your unchanging love, it lets them know they have your support and enables them to heal.

  - **Let them know it'll be okay**

    It is important to let your children know that while things may not be easy, everything will be okay.

  - **Stay close to them**

    Hugging your children often or simply touching them on the shoulder can be looked upon by them as an act of love, and can be very reassuring.

  - **Be honest with your child**

    Honesty is always best, and it's okay to admit that you don't have all of the answers to their concerns.

- **Know when to seek help**

As children go through divorce it is normal for them to display an array of emotions, but they can be healed through love and reassurance. All children are not the same. Some only have a few problems, while for others it is more difficult. If they become overwhelmed it is a sign that it's time to seek professional help.

- **Normal reactions to separation and divorce**

Although strong feelings can be tough on kids, the following reactions can be considered normal for children.

  - Anger
  - Anxiety
  - Mild depression

- **Red flags of a more serious problem**

If your child appears to get worse after a few months, it could be that they are not able to move out of this bout of depression, anxiety, or anger, and need additional help

Some of the warning signs of divorce-related depression or anxiety are:
- ❖ Problems Sleeping
- ❖ Having poor concentration
- ❖ Having trouble at school
- ❖ Falling into drug or alcohol abuse
- ❖ Self-injury, cutting
- ❖ Frequent angry or violent outbursts
- ❖ Withdrawal for loved ones
- ❖ Refusal of loved activities

Discuss these or other signs with your child's doctor, or teachers, or consult a child therapist.

Domestic Violence and Abuse

It is possible for domestic violence and abuse to happen to anyone, but the problem is that it often goes unnoticed, and is dismissed, or denied, and this is normally the case when you're dealing with emotional abuse instead of the physical aspect of abuse. The first step to ending an abusive relationship is recognizing, and admitting that it's taking place. If you or someone you know falls under the guidelines of abuse based on the following warning signs, reach out and tell someone, because living in fear of someone you love isn't something you have to endure.

> **Understanding domestic violence and abuse**

Domestic abuse is also called spousal abuse. It takes place when someone in a live in love relationship, whether it's marriage or dating decides to control the other person, but when this type of abuse involves physical violence, it then becomes what is known as domestic violence. There is only one purpose for domestic violence and abuse, and that is to obtain and keep absolute control over you. Abusers don't play fair, and will use a variety of weapons to wear you down, and keep you under their control such as, fear, guilt, shame, and intimidation. They will also resort to threatening, and hurting both you and those around you.

It is important to note that when it comes to domestic violence and abuse, there is no discrimination. It doesn't matter if the couples are same sex or heterosexual, nor does it matter what your age or ethnicity is, or where you stand in terms of economics. Although this abuse more commonly happens to women, men are also victimized especially when it comes to verbal, and emotional abuse, and though it isn't widely known men also suffer from physical abuse. At the end of the day everyone deserves to be valued, and respected, regardless to whether it is a man, a woman, a teenager, or an elderly person. Abuse is never acceptable on any level or at any time.

➢ **The first step to getting help is identifying the abuse**

Domestic abuse can quickly accelerate from making threats, and doling out verbal abuse to violence. Even though it may appear that physical injury is the most apparent danger, the consequences of emotional abuse are just as severe. Those who endure emotional abuse often end up feeling worthless, helpless, and alone, while suffering from anxiety and depression. This kind of pain shouldn't have to be endured by anyone, and if you want to break free from your situation the first step is recognizing that it is abusive. It is only when you recognize how real your situation is, that you will be able to get the help you need.

➢ **Signs that an abusive relationship exists**

Of the many signs of an abusive relationship, fear of your partner is the most obvious one. Feeling as if you must tread softly around your partner, or be careful of what you say on a consistent basis to avoid an argument, is a sign that you are in an unhealthy and abusive relationship.

➢ **Other signs include:**

- ❖ Being put down by your partner
- ❖ Being controlled by your partner
- ❖ Having self-hatred
- ❖ Feeling helpless
- ❖ Feeling desperate

In answering the questions below, if you have more yes answers than no you are most likely in an abusive relationship.

- ❖ Are you afraid of your partner most of the time?
- ❖ Do you avoid different conversations because it might anger your partner?
- ❖ Do you feel as if nothing that you do for your partner is right?
- ❖ Do you feel as if you deserve to have your partner hurt or mistreat you?
- ❖ Do you ever wonder if you're out of your mind instead of your Partner?
- ❖ Do you feel mentally numb or helpless to do anything?
- ❖ Do you get humiliated and yelled at by your partner?
- ❖ Is your partner very critical of you, and do they belittle you?
- ❖ Are you treated so badly by your partner that you feel embarrassed for your friends or family to see it?
- ❖ Are you sometimes ignored by your partner and belittled because of your opinion or accomplishments?
- ❖ Are you blamed for their abusive behavior?
- ❖ Do you feel like someone's property or a sex object?
- ❖ Is your partner unpredictable with a hot temper?
- ❖ Do they physically abuse you, or say they'll hurt or kill you?
- ❖ Are your children being threatened?
- ❖ Does your partner tell you they'll kill themselves if you leave?
- ❖ Are you forced to have sex with your partner?
- ❖ Are your things being destroyed by them?
- ❖ Do you feel that your partner is possessive of you or that they have a crazy jealous streak?

- ❖ Do they tell you when and where to go?
- ❖ Are you being isolated from your loved ones and friends?
- ❖ Is your money and cell phone use limited?
- ❖ Are you consistently checked up on?

➢ **Domestic violence versus physical abuse**

When speaking of domestic abuse, people are often referencing abuse between spouses or two people in live in relationships. The difference between physical abuse and physical assault is as follows: physical abuse is using bodily force in a way that either injures or put someone in danger. Physical assault, whether it takes place in or out of the family is still a crime, and the police has the ability to protect you from such crimes.

➢ **Sexual abuse is a method of bodily abuse**

Sexual abuse is present in any circumstance where someone is forced to take part in un-consensual sex, unsafe sex, or sexual activities that are degrading. Sex that is forced by someone with whom you also have consensual sex, whether it is a spouse, or someone else you're intimate with is considered to be an act of violence. It is also important to note that there is a higher risk of serious injury, or death for those in relationships with people who abuse them physically and sexually.

➢ **It is still considered abuse if the following occurs**

- ❖ The episodes of physical abuse appear to be minor when you compare them to other occurrences you've seen, or heard about.
- ❖ The occurrences of physical abuse have only taken place once or twice, because if they've done it once the likelihood of the assaults continuing are very good.
- ❖ Once you became passive, and relinquished your right to say what you want to do, where you want to go, and who you wanted to see, the physical assaults ceased. Giving up your rights to keep from being abused doesn't make you victorious.

❖ No physical violence has taken place, but you are still being emotionally, and verbally abused, which can be just as scary, and more confusing to comprehend.

➢ **Emotional abuse**

When thinking of domestic abuse, people usually imagine women who have been beat up, having bruises and scars, however all abusive relationships are not violent ones. The fact that a person isn't beat up doesn't mean they're not suffering from abuse. There are many people, both male and female endure mental abuse which is just as damaging. The unfortunate thing is that, mental abuse is often ignored, even by the one being abused.

➢ **Understanding emotional abuse**

The whole point of emotional abuse is to damage you, causing you to feel worthless and dependent on the abuser. As a victim of emotional abuse, you might feel that you don't have a way out of the relationship, and that you won't have anything unless you are with your abusive partner.

➢ **Examples of emotional abuse includes:**

❖ Yelling

❖ Name calling

❖ Blaming

❖ Making the abused feel shameful

❖ Being isolated

❖ Being controlled

❖ Being intimidated

Those who use emotional abuse will normally threaten acts of violence consequences if you don't do what they say. Many people minimize emotional abuse, thinking that it's not as bad as physical abuse because it doesn't result in a trip to the hospital or leave scars on your body. However emotional scars are quite real, and can be very deeply rooted. As a matter of fact, it is just as damaging as physical abuse, sometimes even more damaging.

➢ **Financial abuse**

Since the abuser's aim is to gain control over you, they will often use money to do so.

➢ **Financial abuse includes**
- ❖ Strictly controlling your money
- ❖ Won't allow you to have money or credit cards
- ❖ Making you tell them what you spend your money on
- ❖ Holding back your basic needs, such as clothing, food, and medicine
- ❖ Giving you an allowance to live on
- ❖ Won't let you work to earn your own money
- ❖ Causing you to miss work or calling your job all of the time
- ❖ Taking all of the money you receive

➢ **The abuser's choice: violent and abusive behavior**

Although many believe people abuse others after losing control of their actions, this is not true. It is actually deliberate or thoughtful actions that are carried out by the abuser in an effort to gain control over you.

➢ **Tactics used by the abuser to manipulate you and exercise their power**

- ❖ **Dominating**

    Because of the need to be in control in the relationship, the abuser will make all of the decisions for the entire family, telling you what you should do, and then expecting you to do it without questioning them, and treating you as a servant, a child or something that belongs to them.

- ❖ **Humiliating**

    The abuser will do whatever is necessary to cause you to look at yourself in a negative fashion or to make you think something is wrong with you. If they can make you feel worthless and that no one else wants you, you probably won't leave. Insulting you, calling you names, and shaming you in public are tactics that are intended to eat away at your self-esteem, and make you feel helpless.

❖ **Isolating**

The abuser wants to cause you to be even more dependent on them, therefore they will try to keep you away from any outside contact, and to do that they will prevent you from seeing family and friends, going to work, or even school. They will also make you ask for their permission before you can do anything, go anywhere, or see anyone.

❖ **Threatening**

In order to get you to drop charges or to keep you from leaving them, the abuser will commonly use threats to scare you. They will threaten to hurt you, your loved ones, or a pet, and even threaten to commit suicide, bring false charges against you, or call child protective services.

❖ **Intimidating**

In order to scare you into submitting the abuser will use different methods to intimidate you, such as giving you threatening looks or signals, breaking things right in front of you, hurting your pets, or showing you weapons, to send the message that there will be violent penalties to pay if you don't do what the say.

❖ **Denying and blaming**

Instead of accepting blame for their actions, the abuser will blame their abusive behavior on having a difficult childhood, a difficult day, or even on the person being abused. They will often try to minimize the abuse or deny that it happened altogether, and will normally shift the blame on to the one being abused.

- **Abusers have the ability to control their behavior**
  - They choose with precision whom they will abuse
  - They are careful about when and where to abuse their victim
  - They can stop abusing at will
  - They usually hit where no evidence is noticeable
  - The cycle of domestic behavior
  - **Abuse**

    The abuser strikes out becoming violent, and putting you down in an effort to show you who the boss is.

  - **Guilt**

    The abuser feels guilty after abusing you, but they're more worried about getting caught and the penalty they will face for what they've done.

  - **Excuses**

    In trying to justify their actions, they drum up a bunch of excuses for what they've done, or blame their victim for their abusive behavior. They'll do anything to avoid responsibility for their behavior.

  - **Normal behavior**

    The abuser will do whatever is necessary to gain control again, in order to keep the person from leaving the relationship. Including acting as if the abuse never took place, or they may even become nice again to give the victim hope that they have sincerely changed.

  - **Fantasy and planning**

    The abuser is now fantasizing about hurting you again. They spend much of their time thinking about the wrong you've done and what they will do to make you pay for it. And then begin creating a plan to turn this fantasy into a reality.

- ❖ **Set-up**

    The abuser begins putting their plan for abusing you to work, where they develop a situation so that they can justify hurting you. Their apologies and gestures of love in between the occurrences of abuse may make it very hard to leave. And they will even trick you into believing no one can help them but you, that this time things will be different, and that they really love you, but if you stay you will continue to be in danger.

➢ **Recognizing the warning signs**

While no one can know everything that goes on behind the doors of someone else's home, there are some telltale signs of domestic abuse and violence that one can look for. And if you see any warning signs in a friend, family member or anyone else you know take them seriously and act on what you see.

➢ **General warning signs**

Abused people may:

- ❖ Appear frightened or eager to please their partner
- ❖ Go along with whatever they say or do
- ❖ Check in with them on a regular basis to let them know where they are and what they're doing.
- ❖ Get harassing phone calls from the partner all day.
- ❖ Make mention of the abuser's jealous temper, or obsession with you

➢ **Warning signs of physical violence**

Those being physically abused may:

- ❖ Be injured but blame it on accidents
- ❖ Be absent from work, school, or family functions with no explanation
- ❖ Put on clothes that will hide any bruises or scars for example, long sleeves while it's hot or sunglasses while inside

➢ **Warning signs of being isolated**

Those being isolated by their abuser may:

- ❖ Not be allowed to see their friends and family
- ❖ Not go out much without their partner
- ❖ Be limited to the amount of money they have, use of credit cards or the car

➢ **Psychological warning signs**

Those being abused may:

- ❖ Have an unusually low self-esteem
- ❖ Appear to have a major change in their personality
- ❖ Become depressed, worried, or suicidal

➢ **What to do if you think someone is being abused**

Speak up if you think someone is being abused. Don't hesitate to do so, by convincing yourself that you should mind your own business, that you could be wrong, or that they probably won't want to talk about it. In letting them know of your concern, it sends the message that you care and could possibly save their life.

➢ **The Do's and Don'ts**

Do

- ❖ Ask if there's a problem
- ❖ Show your concern
- ❖ Listen to what they say and support them
- ❖ Offer your help
- ❖ Back them up in the decisions they make

Don't

- ❖ Wait for them to approach you
- ❖ Be judgmental or blame them for what happened
- ❖ Apply any pressure
- ❖ Give advice unless they ask for it
- ❖ Put stipulations on the support you give

Speak with the person privately and tell them you're concerned. Tell them why you're worried, and that you're there for them whenever they're ready to talk. Set their mind at ease, by letting them know you will keep what they share between the two of you, and make sure they know you will assist them however you can. It is important to remember that people who abuse are quite good at controlling or influencing the person they abuse. When someone has been abused emotionally or physically, they will become depressed, worn down, frightened, shameful, and perplexed. They've been isolated from their family and friends, but need help getting out. By noticing the warning signs and letting them know you'll support them, you may be able to help them get away from an abusive circumstance so they can start healing.

➢ **Places for women to contact for help**

- ❖ In the U.S. call the <u>National Domestic Violence Hotline</u> at 1800-799-7233 (SAFE)
- ❖ In the U.K. call <u>Women's Aid</u> at 0808-2000-247
- ❖ In Australia call 1-800-RESPECT
- ❖ Worldwide: visit <u>The International Directory of Domestic Violence Agencies</u> for a global list of helplines and crisis centers

➢ **Places for men to contact for help**

- ❖ IN U.S. and Canada contact <u>The Domestic Abuse helpline for Men and Women</u> at 1-88-7helpline or 1-888-743-5754

- ❖ In U.K. contact <u>Mankind Initiative</u>
- ❖ In Australia contact <u>One in Three Campaign</u>

Elderly Abuse

Elderly abuse takes place in various places such as in their home, a relative's home and even in the care facilities that are responsible for their cars. If you believe a family member or caregiver is abusing an elderly person, or that they are being taken advantage of financially, please speak up for the sake of that person.

> **What is elderly abuse?**

As elderly people become weaker in their body, their ability to stand up to those who bully, or attack them and fight back becomes lesser and lesser. Their inability to see, hear or think as clearly as they once did, and being limited mentally or physically makes them more vulnerable, and leaves them open to the attack of dishonest people who are waiting to take advantage of them. Many seniors worldwide are subjected to a considerable amount of abuse by those responsible for their care, and in America alone more than 500 million cases of elderly abuse are reported every year, but millions often go unreported.

> **Where elderly abuse takes place**

Elderly abuse generally takes place in he home of the senior, or the abuser that is usually one of their adult children, a grandchild, spouse or the elderly's friend/partner. Abuse also takes place in nursing homes or other home care facilities, especially those that are long-term facilities.

> **Types of elderly abuse**

Elderly abuse occurs in various forms, and they include: intimidation, threats, neglect, and also financial trickery.

Some of the most common types of abuse are:

- ❖ **Physical abuse**

    Any use of force against an elderly person that results in physical pain, a wound, or an injury. Elderly abuse is not limited to bodily assaults such as hitting, but also include improper use of drugs, restraints, or confinement.

- **Emotional abuse**

    Emotional abuse involves talking to or treating an elderly person in ways that causes them psychological pain and include:

    Intimidation through yelling at them or making threats

    Humiliation

    Constant blame or using them as a scapegoat

Types of nonverbal emotional abuse include:

- Ignoring or isolating an elderly person from their friends
- Cutting them off from various activities
- Frightening them
- **Sexual abuse**

    Sexual elder abuse is having sex with an elderly person without their consent. Sexual abuse can include physical sex acts, forcing them to watch sexually graphic material, or other sex acts or forcing them to undress.

- **Neglect or abandonment**

    Neglecting an elderly person, or failing to complete one's obligations as a caregiver, makes up more than one half of all elderly abuse cases that are reported. This neglect can be either intentional or unintentional, due to factors such as one being ignorant of, or denying the fact that an elderly abuse charge needs as much care as they do.

- **Financial manipulation**

    This involves having a caregiver or a scam artist take advantage of an elderly person, by using their money or property without their permission.

Such a person might:

Write checks, use credit cards, or take money out of an elderly's account

    Steal money, monthly checks, or household items

    Sign their signature illegally

    Participate in identity theft

Usual swindles that involve the elderly include:

Telling an elderly person they won a prize, but must pay money to claim it

    Setting up phony charities

    Fraudulent investments

- ❖ Healthcare fraud and abuse

    This type of abuse involves nurses, doctors, and other unethical hospital staff as well as other professional care providers.

Examples of healthcare fraud and abuse include:

Charging for healthcare, but not providing it

    Charging too much or billing twice for medical care services

    Receiving payments for referring people to other providers or writing prescriptions for certain drugs

    Over or under-medicating people

    Recommending different remedies for illnesses or other medical problems that are in fact fraudulent

    Medicaid fraud

➢ **Signs and symptoms of elderly abuse**

Signs of elderly abuse may not be taken seriously or noticeable at first. Some may mistake abuse for dementia, or ill health or this may be what the caregiver will try and lead you to believe it is. Although some of the signs and symptoms of elderly abuse may resemble indications of a declining memory, don't dismiss them based solely upon what the caregiver says, but instead investigate further.

➢ **General signs of abuse**

General types of elderly abuse include:

- ❖ Regular arguments taking place between the elderly person and their caregiver
- ❖ Personality or behavioral changes

If you think and elderly person is being abused, but you're not sure, check for groups of the following signs in their behavior or physically.

➢ **Physical abuse**

- ❖ Having a series of unexplained injuries such as black eyes, bruises, or scratches, especially if they appear evenly on both sides of the body.
- ❖ Fractured bones, or sprained wrists/ankles
- ❖ Drug overdoses being reported or having more medicine left than they should because it's not being taken
- ❖ Broken eyeglasses
- ❖ Signs that they are being tied down, such as marks on the wrist from ropes
- ❖ Caregiver will not allow anyone to see the person alone

➢ **Emotional abuse**

Other signs of emotional elderly abuse include:

- ❖ Witnessing threats, put downs, or controlling behavior from a caregiver
- ❖ The actions of the elderly person, resembles signs of dementia, such as rocking back and forth, sucking, or muttering to oneself.

➢ **Sexual abuse**

- ❖ Bruised breasts or sex organs
- ❖ Mysterious STD's or genital infections

- ❖ Mysterious bleeding from the vagina or anus
- ❖ Under wear that's been stained, torn or has blood on them

➢ **Caregiver neglect or self-neglect**
- ❖ Losing too much weight, not eating enough, not enough water
- ❖ Bed sores or other medical conditions that goes untreated
- ❖ Filthy living conditions: dirty, bugs in the house, dirty sheets and clothing
- ❖ Not clean or not bathing
- ❖ Not dressed properly for the weather conditions
- ❖ House in dangerous condition (heat not on, no running water, electrical problems or other hazards)
- ❖ Being left stranded at a public place

➢ **Being financially exploited**
- ❖ Drawing a lot of money from an elderly person's account
- ❖ Financial conditions have changed suddenly
- ❖ Money and other belongings missing from the elderly's home
- ❖ Will and power of attorney, house title, or insurance policy was changed
- ❖ Other names being added to senior's signature card on bank account
- ❖ Elder has enough money but lacks medical care and bills aren't being paid
- ❖ Elderly person can't walk, or leave home, but money has been taken from ATM, or bank
- ❖ Things that the elderly person doesn't need are being bought

➢ **Healthcare fraud and abuse**
- ❖ More than one bills for same medical service or device such as a phone
- ❖ Person is showing signs of getting either too much medicine or not enough

- ❖ Signs that elder isn't being cared for properly even though bills are paid in full
- ❖ Person is receiving poor care from elderly care facility: people not trained right, or not paid enough, facility is crowded, concerns are going unanswered

➢ **Risk factors for elderly abuse**

Caring for an elderly person with a lot of different needs that have to be met, and being an elderly person who have lost their independence, and also have health issues is difficult. Each situation can create circumstances under which the elderly person is likely to be abused.

➢ **Risk factors concerning caregivers**

While it can be very satisfying and inspiring for family members to care for an elderly relative, the responsibilities and demands of caring for them can become quite overwhelming, as the elderly person's health begins to decline. The stress of such care can cause the caregiver to have mental and physical issues that may trigger the caregiver to become stressed, and impatient which may in turn cause them to lash out at the elderly person.

When dealing with caregivers the significant risk factors include:

- ❖ Being unable to deal with stress
- ❖ Depressed
- ❖ Insufficient support from other possible caregivers
- ❖ Caregiver acts as if the senior is a burden, and caring for them is unrewarding
- ❖ Caregiver uses drugs

Even if a caregiver works in a nursing home or other institutional settings, their level of stress due to a lack of training, too much responsibility, working in unsuitable conditions, or not having the personality or character needed for their line of work can lead to elderly abuse.

➤ The condition and history of the elderly

Even though nothing can excuse abuse, there are several factors concerning the elderly person themselves that can sometimes determine whether the risk of being abused is greater, and they are:

- ❖ How sick they are or how far along their dementia is
- ❖ Being stuck alone with the caregiver for long periods of time
- ❖ The elderly person was once an abusive parent or spouse
- ❖ There was once domestic violence in the home
- ❖ The elderly person is verbally abusive and they are physically aggressive

In many cases just because a caregiver may abuse, it's not necessarily because they intend to, but it may be because they have exceeded their capabilities, and have become overwhelmed.

➤ Preventing abuse

There are three things that can be done to prevent elderly abuse:

- ❖ Listen to both the elderly and the caregiver
- ❖ Get involved if you think abuse is taking place
- ❖ Teach others how to identify and report elder abuse

➤ What can a caregiver do to prevent abuse?

If the demands of caring for an elderly person overwhelms you, do these things:

- ❖ Ask your family and friends or local agencies for help, so that you can get a break even if it's only for two hours
- ❖ Seek out an adult daycare facility
- ❖ Take care of your health
- ❖ If you begin feeling depressed get help, if not it could lead to abuse
- ❖ Look for a support group or caregivers of seniors
- ❖ If you are a substance abuser get help

If you think you might possibly cross the line, keep in mind that calling an elderly abuse helpline can enable you to get the support you need. So pick up the phone and call.

➢ **As a concerned relative or friend what can you do?**
- ❖ Look for warning signs, and if you think abuse is happening report it
- ❖ Keep an eye on their medicine. Check the date and amount to see if they are taking the required amount
- ❖ Keep an eye on their finances, and ask for permission to look at bank accounts and credit card statements. Look for inconsistencies
- ❖ Keep in touch, and visit regularly
- ❖ Volunteer to give the caregiver a break. If possible, do it on a regular basis

➢ **How to protect you as an elderly from abuse**
- ❖ If your finances are not in order get professional help or talk to someone you can trust to help you
- ❖ Don't isolate yourself from family and friends. Keep in touch.
- ❖ If you feel you're being abused or your care is insufficient, and you're not happy it doesn't matter where you're being cared for, tell someone you can trust and ask if they will call the abuse hotline for you.

If you are not able to help an elderly person there are many other things you can do to assist in other ways, such as volunteering, donating money to educate other's about elderly abuse, and lobbying for stronger laws and policies.

➢ **Reporting abuse**

Don't take for granted that someone else will help the person that you suspect of being abused or that they can help their self, this is not necessarily true. Many times seniors won't report abuse for reasons such as fear of retaliation, or they think they won't have anyone else to care for them if they turn their caregiver in to the authorities. If by chance the caregiver is one of their children, they could be embarrassed or ashamed of the fact or blame themselves. Or they may be trying to protect their child.

- ➢ **How to report elderly abuse**

The first place you should contact is **APS** or **Adult Protective Services.** They investigate abuse cases, get involved, and offer their services or advice, but the power and scope of services vary from state to state. Some important things to remember when reporting elderly abuse to make sure you are able to give the information clearly and accurately are:

- ❖ **Try and be as specific as possible when giving your description**
- ❖ **Remember that the elder has a right to refuse the help or services you enlist**
- ❖ **Keep both your eyes and ears open at all times**

- ➢ **Reporting and stopping elderly abuse**

State Directory of Helplines, Hotlines, and Elder Abuse Prevention Resources - National Center on Elder Abuse

- ❖ U.S: 1800-677-1116 (Elder locator)
- ❖ UK: 0808 808 8141 or Ireland: 1800 940 010 (Action on Elder Abuse)
- ❖ Australia: 1300 651 192 (Elder Abuse Prevention Unit)
- ❖ South Africa: 080 111 2131 (Age In Action)
- ❖ Canada: visit Alberta Elder Abuse for links to resources

Stress

In this modern society we live in, life is filled with troubles, goals that must be met, hindrances, and also stressful demands and for a lot of people stress is so normal that it has become a way of life with them, but it isn't always bad. Stress can be helpful when working under pressure, and at times can inspire you to do your best when it comes in limited doses. But if you're consistently living your life in crisis mode, both the mind and body will be greatly affected. However, if you are able to identify the signs and symptoms of stress, and take the necessary precautions to lessen its harmful affects, you can protect yourself.

➢ What is stress?

Stress is a typical fleshly response, to events that cause you to feel endangered or disturbs your sense of balance in some sort of way. Whenever someone senses a threat, it doesn't matter if it's real or imaginary, the body's defenses automatically accelerate into high gear which is known as the stress response, and is the body's way of protecting itself. If your stress response is working properly, it will help you to maintain your focus, remain energized, and vigilant, and if an emergency should arise it can even save your life, by affording you additional strength to protect yourself. In addition, the stress response can also help you rise to the occasion if you will, to face new challenges. Stress works to your advantage at times, for example, it helps you stay on top of things during a work presentation, helps to hone or sharpen your focus when taking a test, or pushes you to study for a test when you would much rather do something else. But when it reaches a certain point, it ceases being an asset, and begins causing great harm to your health, your frame of mind, your ability to produce, your relationships, and also the quality of life you lead.

➢ The Body's Stress Response

Whenever a person senses a threat an influx of stress hormones, such as adrenaline and cortisol are released from the nervous system, serving to incite the body to act in times of a crisis. As this takes place, your heart begins to beat faster, your muscles get tighter, your blood pressure elevates, you begin breathing at a faster pace, and your mind becomes clearer. These physical alterations give your more strength and endurance, causes you to react quicker, and improves your concentration, thus preparing you to either fight or run away from the danger you're facing.

➢ How to respond to stress

Being able to recognize when your stress levels are out of control is very important, because of the fact that it creeps up on you with great ease, and this the most dangerous aspect of stress. Before long you begin to get used to it, it becomes very familiar for you, and even normal, so much so that you don't realize just how great it's affecting you, even as it begins to take a greater toll.

There is no one sign or symptom that helps you identify when you're on stress overload, because it can be just about anything. There are many different ways in which stress can affect one's mind, body, and behavior and not everyone has the same signs and symptoms. A tremendous amount of stress not only leads to dangerous mental and physical health issues, but it will also affect all of your relationships, whether it is at work, home, or school.

➢ Stress doesn't necessarily look stressful

One psychologist uses an analogy for driving a vehicle, to describe the three most common methods people use to respond when overcome by stress, and they are:

❖ Foot on the gas peddle

This stress response is one where you are irate, irritated, or ready to fight. You become fired up, filled with intense anger, extremely emotional, and lack the ability to sit still.

❖ Foot on the brake peddle

This stress response is one where you are withdrawn, depressed, or want to run away. You will totally shut down, pull away from people, become zoned out, and display little or no energy or emotions.

❖ Foot on both peddles

This stress response is one where you simply become tense, or freeze up. When under pressure, you become frozen and can't do anything. You have a paralyzed look on your face, but deep down you are tremendously disturbed.

➢ Stress overload signs and symptoms

The following is a list of common warning signs and symptoms of stress. The more of these that you recognize within yourself, the sooner you may go into stress overload.

- ❖ **Cognitive symptoms**
  - Memory loss
  - No ability to focus
  - Lacking proper judgment
  - Being very pessimistic
  - Anxiety
  - Always worrying
- ❖ **Emotional symptoms**
  - Moody
  - Irritable
  - Agitated, can't relax
  - Overwhelmed
  - Feeling lonely and isolated
  - Depressed
- ❖ **Physical symptoms**
  - Aches and pain
  - Diarrhea or constipated
  - Nauseated
  - Pain in the chest or heart palpitations
  - No sexual desires
  - Catching colds on a consistent basis
- ❖ **Behavioral symptoms**
  - Inconsistent eating habit
  - Inconsistent sleeping habits
  - Becoming isolated from others

- Procrastination
- Drinking, smoking, or using drugs
- Nervous habits (e.g. nail biter)

It is important to note that the signs and symptoms of stress can also be related to other emotional or medical issues. So if you're feeling any stress related signs and symptoms, it is vital for you to go to your doctor for a full assessment, to determine if your symptoms are related to stress.

➢ **What is considered too much stress?**

Stress, can do a phenomenal amount of damage therefore it is vital to know how much you can handle. So the question we need to ask is, how much stress is too much, because when it comes to how much stress one can handle, everyone is different. There are some who can handle stress with no problem at all, and then there are those who seem to fall apart while facing even the smallest of hindrances. And amazingly so, some people appear to be able to flourish on the pleasure and trials of a highly stressful lifestyle. A person's ability to cope with stress depends upon many different aspects, which includes how fruitful your relationships are, how positive or negative you might think, what type of emotional intelligence you have, and also your genetic makeup.

➢ **That which influences your stress tolerance level**

❖ **A strong support network**

When you have a strong network of family and friends who support you, this can be a huge safeguard against those things in life that causes you stress. But the flip side of the coin is that the more isolated you remain, the more open you will be to stress.

❖ **Your sense of control**

If you have self-confidence as well as an assurance of your ability to impact the events you face, and endure the challenges you're confronted with, it may be easier to cope with your stress. But if you sense that those events are spinning out of control, you will have a lower tolerance for stress.

❖ **Your attitude and outlook**

Those who are optimistic often handle stress better. They are able to accept challenge they have a great sense of humor, and embraces the fact that change is a part of life.

❖ **Your ability to cope with your emotions**

If you don't understand how to soothe and relax yourself when you're experiencing feelings of sadness, and anger, or that you are being overcome by your circumstances, you will be tremendously vulnerable to stress. The ability to bounce back from a hardship depends on whether or not you can bring your emotions under control, and this is a skill that can be learned no matter what your age is.

❖ **Your knowledge and preparation**

If you know as much as there is to know about a stressful situation, including how long it will last, it will be easier for you to cope with. For example, if you go into a shelter with your children with a realistic view of what to expect in the interim, the trials of living under those circumstances will be less traumatic for you than it would be, if you were expecting to find a place to live immediately.

❖ **Causes of stress**

The circumstances and burdens that trigger stress are known as stressors, which we normally see as something negative, such as a grueling work schedule or a bad relationship. But truthfully, anything that puts a great burden on you can be stressful. This can be positive events such as planning a wedding, purchasing a home, going off to college in a different state, or getting a job promotion. All stress isn't triggered by outward influences that can be seen or noticed by others, for example, if you're the type that worry too much about things that may or may not take place, or you have unrealistic, or negative thoughts about life, this can really stress you out, because what triggers stress is partly contingent, on how you see it. Something that stresses you out may not affect the next person at all. In fact, they might even enjoy it. For example, your commute to a job interview might cause you to be nervous, and irritated because you feel the traffic is too heavy and you might be late, but someone else may be very relaxed because they left early enough to have more than enough time, and love listening to a particular radio station while they drive.

- **Common outward influences that cause stress**
  - Major changes in life
  - Money problems
  - Work
  - A heavy schedule
  - Problematic relationships
  - Family and children

- **Common inward influences that cause stress**
  - Being a chronic worrier
  - Being a negative thinker/pessimistic
  - Saying negative things about oneself
  - Having unrealistic expectations of oneself
  - Having no flexibility, too hard on oneself
  - Having an all-or-nothing attitude

- **Effects of chronic stress**

The body has no way of determining whether a threat is physical or psychological. It doesn't matter what you're stressing over, it could be a very full schedule, an argument, an excessive amount of bills, or you could be stuck in traffic, your body will respond the same as it would if your life was in danger. When you are on stress overload your emergency stress response will probably be on most of the time, and the more it is activated, it becomes harder and harder to shut it off.

Chronic stress, can interfere with pretty much every system in the body, and when coping with stress for long periods of time it can cause serious health issues, such as high blood pressure, a low immune system, heart attack, stroke, infertility, and speeding up the aging process. It can even cause one's brain to be rewired, leaving them more open to anxiety and depression.

➢ **Some of the health issues that are caused by stress include:**
- ❖ Various kinds of pain
- ❖ Heart disease
- ❖ Depression
- ❖ Weight issues
- ❖ Digestive issues
- ❖ Autoimmune diseases
- ❖ Sleeping problems
- ❖ Skin conditions, such as eczema

➢ **Dealing with the symptoms of stress**

Stress, that is allowed to go on without being treated can be quite harmful, but one generally has a greater ability to control their stress levels than they think they do. Although they may not realize it, many people in an effort to cope with their stress, use methods that only add to the problem. For example, when trying to unwind at the end of a stressful day, they might drink too much, eat large amounts of food, spend too many hours in front of the TV or computer, use medicine to relax, or strike out at other people. There are many different methods of dealing with stress and its symptoms that are healthier. Everyone's stress response is different, and there is no one solution that works for everyone or every situation, so you may need to try different techniques and focus on what helps you feel free from stress and in more control.

> **Learning how to cope with stress**

Even though it seems like the things that are stressing you is out of control, you have total control over the way you respond to them. When dealing with your stress, it is simply about being in control of your thoughts, emotions, schedule, environment, and how you cope with your problems. Managing your stress consists of changing the things that stresses you out, changing how you react to them when you can't change things, giving yourself the proper care you deserve, and taking the time to relax and get your proper rest.

There are four things you need to remember and they are: **Avoid, Alter, Adapt,** or **Accept**.

- **Avoid** stress that's not necessary.

    Although you can't avoid all stress, learning to say no, determining which things on your to-do list should be done, versus that which must be done, and staying away from people and situations that stress you out. This can help you eliminate a lot of your daily stressors.

- **Alter** the situation that brings on stress.

    If a situation can't be avoided, try and alter it. Be firm and confront your problems head on. Rather than suppressing your feelings, and allowing your stress to build up, in a respectful manner, share your concerns with others. Or at least be willing to find a half way mark and work the issue out.

- **Adapt** to the stressor.

    If you don't have the ability to change the stressor, work on changing yourself, by restructuring the problem or concentrating on the positive things in your life. If a part of your job is stressing you, concentrate on an area of your job that you really enjoy. Focus on the big picture, and ask yourself if it is truly something that is worth getting upset over.

- ❖ **Accept** what you can't change.

    For as long as you live, there will be stressors that you can't do anything about. But instead of being critical of the situation, and causing even more stress, learn to accept what you can't change. Look for the good in every circumstance, because even the situations that are most stressful can be an opportunity for you to learn or grow. Lastly, learn to accept the fact that no one will ever be perfect, not even you.

    Strengthening your physical health will also help you deal with the symptoms of stress.

- ❖ **Set aside time to relax**
- ❖ **Get regular exercise**
- ❖ **Practice eating healthy**
- ❖ **Get your proper sleep**

Managing stress isn't always enough. If you have an overwhelming sense of stress, and don't feel as if you can o through with the stress management program, it's possible you might need some extra help.

There are two core skills that are good for reducing overwhelming stress, and they are:

- ❖ **Quick stress relief**

    Using your senses such as what you see, taste, touch, hear and smell, or simply through movement is the best method of quickly reducing stress. Some methods you can use to quickly relax yourself are: looking a favorite photograph, smelling a particular scent, listening to a favorite song, tasting your favorite food, or hugging someone you really love. Everyone won't respond to these sensory experiences in the same manner. What may relax one person may totally irritate someone else. But experimenting with your senses will help you determine the sensory experience that best suits you.

❖ **Emotional connection**

Being emotionally detached from oneself and others will contribute more to chronic stress than anything else, and learning to understand the affect your emotions have on your thoughts and actions is important when it comes to dealing with your stress. You don't have to live life as if on a rollercoaster ride with crazy ups and downs. When you finally become aware of your emotions, even the ones that cause the most pain, which you try to suppress, the easier it will be for you to understand your own motivations. You will also be able to stop saying or doing things that you will regret later on, and gain a renewed sense of energy.

Once you are able to fully grasp these core skills you will be able to confront your stressful challenges confidently, knowing that you will be armed with the ability to bring yourself back into balance very quickly.

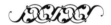

GLOSSARY

Abandonment - The relinquishment or renunciation of an interest, claim, privilege, possession, or right, especially with the intent of never again resuming or reasserting it.

Abandoned child syndrome - A behavioral or psychological condition that results from the loss of one or both parents. Abandonment may be physical (the parent is not present in the child's life) or emotional (the parent withholds affection, nurturing, or stimulation

Abusive behavior - A general term for various behaviors which may be aggressive, coercive or controlling, destructive, harassing, intimidating, isolating, or threatening, that a batterer or abuser may use to control a domestic partner, child or other victim.

Acid reflux - A chronic symptom of mucosal damage caused by stomach acid coming up from the stomach into the esophagus.

Acomprosate - A drug used for treating alcohol and benzodiazepine dependence.

Addiction – A strong and harmful need to regularly have something, such as a drug or do something, such as gamble.

Addictive – Causing a strong and harmful need to regularly have or do something.

Adult protective services - Social services provided to abused, neglected, or exploited older adults and adults with significant disabilities. APS is typically administered by local or state health, aging, or regulatory departments and includes a multidisciplinary approach to helping older adults, and younger adults with disabilities that are victims.

Affordable Care Act - A United States federal statute signed into law by President Barack Obama on March 23, 2010. The ACA was enacted with the goals of increasing the quality and affordability of health insurance, lowering the uninsured rate by expanding public and private insurance coverage, and reducing the costs of healthcare for individuals and the government.

Agoraphobia - An anxiety disorder characterized by anxiety in situations where the sufferer perceives certain environments as dangerous or uncomfortable, often due to the environment's vast openness or crowdedness.

AIDS - A disease of the human immune system that is characterized cytologically especially by a reduction in the numbers of CD4-bearing helper T cells to 20 percent or less of normal thereby rendering the subject highly vulnerable to life-threatening conditions (as Pneumocystis carinii pneumonia) and to some that become life threatening (as Kaposi's sarcoma) and that is caused by infection with HIV commonly transmitted in infected blood especially during illicit intravenous drug use and in bodily secretions (as semen) during sexual intercourse.

Alcohol abuse - A psychiatric diagnosis describing the recurring use of alcohol despite its negative consequences.

Alcohol dependence - A substance-related disorder in which an individual is physically or psychologically dependent upon drinking alcohol.

Alcoholics anonymous - An international fellowship of men and women who have had a drinking problem.

Alcoholism – A medical condition in which someone frequently drinks too much and becomes unable to live a normal and healthy life.

Altercation – An angry or heated discussion or quarrel; argument.

Amphetamine - A racemic sympathomimetic amine $C_9H_{13}N$ or one of its derivatives, such as dextroamphetamine or methamphetamine frequently abused as a stimulant of the central nervous system but used clinically especially in the form of its sulfate $C_9H_{13}N \cdot H_2SO_4$ to treat attention deficit disorder and narcolepsy and formerly as a short-term appetite suppressant.

Amygdala - A roughly almond-shaped mass of gray matter inside each cerebral hemisphere, involved with the experiencing of emotions.

Anabolic steroids - Any of a group of usually synthetic hormones that are derivatives of testosterone, are used medically especially to promote tissue growth, and are sometimes abused by athletes to increase the size and strength of their muscles and improve endurance.

Analgesia - Insensibility to pain without loss of consciousness.

Angel dust - Commonly known as **PCP** and known colloquially as **Angel Dust** and many other names, is a recreational dissociative drug.

Anorexia nervosa - A psychiatric disorder characterized by an unrealistic fear of weight gain, self-starvation, and conspicuous distortion of body image.

Anorexic - A person with anorexia nervosa.

Anti-anxiety medicine - Any of a class of drugs that reduce anxiety, such as tranquilizers.

Anti-depressant – Medication used or tending to relieve or prevent psychic depression.

Anti-psychotic medicine - Any antipsychotic drug, such as chlorpromazine: used to treat such conditions as schizophrenia.

Anti-social behavior – Displaying violent and harmful behavior toward people.

Anti-social personality disorder – A personality disorder that is characterized by antisocial behavior, exhibiting pervasive disregard for and violation of the rights, feelings and safety of others starting in childhood or the early teenage years, and continuing into adulthood, also called psychopathic personality disorder.

Attention deficit hyperactive disorder (ADHD) – A psychiatric disorder or neurobehavioral disorder characterized by significant difficulties, either of inattention and/or hyperactivity and impulsiveness.

Anxiety attack - A sudden acute episode of intense anxiety and feelings of panic attack.

Anxiety disorder – An umbrella term that covers several forms of a type of common psychiatric disorder, characterized by excessive rumination, worrying, uneasiness, apprehension, and fear about future uncertainties either based on real or imagined events. Which may affect both physical and psychological health.

Asperger's syndrome - An autism spectrum disorder (ASD) that is characterized by significant difficulties in social interaction and nonverbal communication, alongside restricted and repetitive patterns of behavior and interests.

Autism – A complex developmental disorder distinguished by difficulties with social interaction, verbal and nonverbal communication, and behavioral problems, including repetitive behaviors and narrow focus of interest.

Autoimmune disease - The failure of an organism in recognizing its own constituent parts as *self*, which allows an immune response against its own cells and tissues.

Barbiturates - Any of various derivatives of barbituric acid (as phenobarbital) that are used especially as sedatives, hypnotics, and antispasmodics and are often addictive.

Behavioral symptoms - Observable manifestations of impaired psychological functioning.

Benzodiazepines - A class of psychoactive drugs whose core chemical structure is the fusion of a benzene ring and a diazepine ring.

Binge – A period of excessive or uncontrolled indulgence in food or drink.

Binge eating cycle - A vicious cycle in which those with binge eating disorder eat to feel better, feel even worse for eating, and then turn back to food for more relief.

Binge eating disorder - Compulsive overeating in which people consume huge amounts of food while feeling out of control and powerless to stop.

Biological – Of, relating to, caused by, or affecting life or living organisms: biological processes such as growth and digestion.

Bipolar disorder – A psychiatric disorder marked by alternating episodes of mania and depression, also called bipolar illness, manic-depressive illness.

Body's stress response – The body's response in a time of crisis, when a person senses a threat, causing an influx of stress hormones such as adrenaline, and cortisol to be released from the nervous system.

Borderline personality disorder – A personality disorder marked by a long standing pattern of instability in interpersonal relationships, behavior, mood, and self-image that can interfere with, social or occupational functioning or cause extreme emotional distress.

Brain chemistry - The study of the chemical composition and processes of the nervous system and the effects of chemicals on it.

Bulimia Nervosa - An eating disorder, common especially among young women of normal or nearly normal weight, that is characterized by episodic binge eating and followed by feelings of guilt, depression, and self-condemnation. It is often associated with measures taken to prevent weight gain, such as self-induced vomiting, the use of laxatives, dieting, or fasting.

Bulimic - A person suffering from bulimia.

Buprenorphine - A semisynthetic narcotic analgesic that is derived from thebaine and is administered in the form of its hydrochloride $C_{29}H_{41}NO_4 \cdot HCl$ intravenously or intramuscularly to treat moderate to severe pain and sublingually to treat opioid dependence.

Caregiver burnout stress – A condition of exhaustion, anger, rage, or guilt that results from unrelieved caring for a chronically ill dependent. Health care professionals often use the term but it is not listed in the Diagnostic and Statistical Manual of Mental Disorders.

Carbamazepine – An anticonvulsant and analgesic drug used in the treatment of certain forms of epilepsy and to relieve pain associated with trigeminal neuralgia.

Carpal tunnel syndrome – A disorder caused by compression at the wrist of the median nerve supplying the hand, causing numbness and tingling.

Catastrophic - Extremely harmful; bringing physical or financial ruin.

Celibacy – A state of being unmarried and abstinent from sexual relations.

Celibate – Referring to one who abstains from sexual intercourse.

Checkers – People who suffer with OCD that check things over and over, that they connect with being injured or put in danger.

Chemical messenger - Any compound that serves to transmit a message, and may refer to:

Hormone- Long range chemical messenger, Neurotransmitter- communicates to adjacent cells,

Neuropeptide- a protein sequence which acts as a hormone or neurotransmitter, Pheromone- a chemical factor that triggers a social response in members of the same species.

Child abuse and neglect - Any recent act or failure to act on the part of a parent or caretaker which results in death, serious physical or emotional harm, sexual abuse or exploitation, an act or failure to act which presents an imminent risk of serious harm.

Chronic stress - The response to emotional pressure suffered for a prolonged period over which an individual perceives he or she has no control.

Citalopram – An antidepressant compound used in the treatment of major depressive disorder.

Cocaine - A tropane alkaloid that is obtained from the leaves of the coca plant. It is addictive due to its effect on the mesolimbic reward pathway.

Cognitive-behavioral therapy – An action-oriented form of psychosocial therapy that assumes that maladaptive, or faulty thinking patterns cause maladaptive behavior and negative emotions. (Maladaptive behavior is counter-productive or interferes with everyday life).

Compulsion - An irresistible impulse to act, regardless of the rationality of the motivation.

Compulsive behavior - Defined as performing an act persistently and repetitively without it necessarily leading to an actual reward or pleasure.

Compulsive eaters – Someone with an eating disorder characterized by continuous or frequent excessive eating over which an individual does not feel he or she has control, and which usually leads to weight gain and obesity.

Compulsive internet use – Characterized by an excessive use of computers or other devices, e.g. smartphones, tablet-pcs etc., for online activities, to an extent that other activities of daily life are severely compromised.

Compulsive gambling - The uncontrollable urge to keep gambling despite the toll it takes on your life.

Computer addiction - The excessive or compulsive use of the computer, which persists despite the serious negative consequences for personal, social or occupational function.

Coping skills - The skills that we use to offset disadvantages in day-to-day life. Coping skills can be seen as a sort of adaptation, such as the finely tuned hearing that many visually impaired people develop.

Counters and arrangers – Those suffering with OCD that must have everything in a specific arrangement, and it must be in equal numbers.

Counter productive - Tending to hinder or act against the achievement of a goal.

Cutting - A form of repetitive self-injury in which a person deliberately cuts the skin, as to cope with stress or negative emotions.

Cyber addiction - The problematic use of the Internet, including the various aspects of its technology, such as electronic mail (e-mail) and the World Wide Web.

Cyber relationship - A form of interpersonal communication, often including intimate relationships between people who have met over the internet.

Cyber relationship addiction - The addiction to social networking in all forms.

Cyber sex - A form of long-distance eroticism in which one's sexual fantasies are relayed to another participant in a real-time computer chat forum, who may self-stimulate himself/herself to a point of sexual gratification

Cyber sex addiction - people addict to social networking, chat rooms or messaging on online

Decreased libido – A decreased sex drive.

Delayed orgasm - The inability or failure to experience orgasm.

Delusions - Idiosyncratic false beliefs that are firmly maintained in spite of incontrovertible and obvious proof or evidence to the contrary.

Dementia - A loss of mental ability severe enough to interfere with normal activities of daily living, lasting more than six months, not present since birth, and not associated with a loss or alteration of

Demerol - A narcotic pain medicine used to treat moderate to severe pain.

Dependent personality disorder – A persistent mental state characterized by a lack of self-confidence and an inability to function independently.

Depressant - A drug or endogenous compound that lowers neurotransmission levels, which is to depress or reduce arousal or stimulation, in various areas of the brain. Depressants are also occasionally referred to as "downers" as they lower the level of arousal when taken.

Depression – A mental state of altered mood characterized by feelings of sadness, despair, and discouragement.

Desensitization - Treatment of phobias and related disorders by intentionally exposing the patient, in imagination or in real life, to a hierarchy of emotionally distressing stimuli.

Detoxification - The physiological or medicinal removal of toxic substances from a living organism, including, but not limited to, the human body and additionally can refer to the period of withdrawal during which an organism returns to homeostasis after long-term use of an addictive substance.

Developmental disorders - A form of mental retardation that develops in some children after they have progressed normally for the first 3 or 4 years of life.

Dialectical behavioral therapy - A therapy designed to help people change patterns of behavior that are not effective, such as self-harm, suicidal thinking and substance abuse.

Dilaudid - A narcotic pain reliever used to treat moderate to severe pain.

Disorganized behavior – The lack of ability to care for oneself, work a job, have a conversation with or do things with other people

Disorganized speech – Fragmented thinking, which hinders the ability to focus, and maintain a train of thought.

Diuretics - A substance or drug that tends to increase the discharge of urine.

Divalproex sodium - An anticonvulsant used in the treatment of petit mal and related seizure disorders.

Domestic violence and abuse - A pattern of abusive behavior in any relationship that is used by one partner to gain or maintain power and control over another intimate partner.

Dopamine - A hormone and neurotransmitter of the catecholamine and phenethylamine families that plays a number of important roles in the human brain and body.

Doubters and sinners – Those suffering from schizophrenia that fear, if they don't do everything perfect, something bad will happen to them.

Dry eyes – Characterized by decreased tear flow and thickening and hardening of the cornea and conjunctiva.

Dysfunction - The condition of having poor and unhealthy behaviors and attitudes within a group of people. Medical: the state of being unable to function in a normal way.

Dysthymia - A form of chronic unipolar depression that tends to occur in elderly persons with debilitating physical disorders, multiple interpersonal losses, and chronic marital difficulties.

Eating Disorders Anonymous - A fellowship of individuals who share their experience, strength and hope with each other that they may solve their common problems and help others to recover from their eating disorders.

E-cigarette - A battery-powered vaporizer that has the feel of tobacco smoking. They produce a mist rather than cigarette smoke

Ecstasy - A empathogenic drug of the phenethylamine and amphetamine classes of drugs. Also known as MDMA, it increases a sense of intimacy and diminishes anxiety with others that can induce euphoria and mild psychedelia.

Elderly abuse - Also called elder mistreatment, senior abuse, abuse in later life, abuse of older adults, abuse of older women, and abuse of older men, it is a single, or repeated act, or lack of appropriate action, occurring within any relationship where there is an expectation of trust, which causes harm or distress to an older person.

Emotional abuse - A form of abuse characterized by a person subjecting or exposing another to behavior that may result in psychological trauma, including anxiety, chronic depression, or post-traumatic stress disorder.

Emotional and psychological trauma - The result of extraordinarily stressful events that shatter your sense of security, making you feel helpless and vulnerable in a dangerous world.

Emotional stress - A person's response to a stressor such as an environmental condition or a stimulus

Euphoria - A feeling of well being or elation; especially: one that is groundless, disproportionate to its cause, or inappropriate to one's life situation.

Equilibrium - The condition of a system in which all competing influences are balanced, in a wide variety of contexts.

Escalation - The process of increasing or rising, derived from the concept of an escalator.

Escitaloprom - An antidepressant of the selective serotonin reuptake inhibitor (SSRI) class. The U.S. Food, and Drug Administration have approved it for the treatment of adults and children over 12 years of age with major depressive disorder and generalized anxiety disorder.

Exhibitionism - The act or practice of behaving so as to attract attention to oneself.

Eye movement desensitization and reprocessing or EDMR- A psychotherapy that emphasizes disturbing memories as the cause of psychopathology, and alleviates the symptoms of post-traumatic stress disorder. EMDR is used for individuals who have experienced severe trauma that remains unresolved.

Fetishism - The pathological displacement of erotic interest and satisfaction to a fetish.

Financial abuse - Telling you what you can and cannot buy or requiring you to share control of your bank accounts.

Financial exploitation - Illegal or improper use of an elder's funds, property, or assets.

Financial manipulation - Deliberately deceiving the victim with the promise of goods, services, or other benefits that are nonexistent, unnecessary, never intended to be provided, or grossly misrepresented.

Fluoxetine - A drug that functions as an SSRI, and is administered in the form of its hydrochloride $C_{17}H_{18}F_3NO \cdot HCl$ especially to treat depression, panic disorder, and obsessive-compulsive disorder.

Fluvoxamine - A drug that functions as an SSRI and is administered orally, especially to treat depression and obsessive-compulsive disorder.

Frontal lobe - The anterior division of each cerebral hemisphere having its lower part in the anterior fossa of the skull and bordered behind by the central sulcus.

Gallbladder disease - A term for several types of conditions that can affect your gallbladder, a small pear shaped sac located under the liver. Your gallbladder's main function is to store the bile produced in your liver and pass it along to the small intestine.

Gamblers anonymous - A fellowship of men and women who share their experience, strength and hope with each other that they may solve their common problem and help others to recover from a gambling problem.

Gastrointestinal issues – Problems with food digestion.

Generalized anxiety disorder - An anxiety disorder that is characterized by excessive, uncontrollable and often irrational worry about everyday things that is disproportionate to the actual source of worry.

Gooseflesh - A pimply state of the skin with the hairs erect, produced by cold or fright.

Grandeur - Splendor and impressiveness, especially of appearance or style.

Group support - The act of supporting or the condition of being supported by a group of people.

Group therapy - The (methods of) treatment of disease, disorders of the body *etc.*, in a group setting.

Hallucinogenic substances - A psychoactive agent which can cause hallucinations, perception anomalies, and other substantial subjective changes in thoughts, emotion, and consciousness.

Hallucinations - A perception of something, such as a visual image or a sound with no external cause usually arising from a disorder of the nervous system or in response to drugs, such as LSD.

Healthy sex behavior - Is defined as: Enjoyment of sexual relation without exploitation, oppression or abuse, safe pregnancy and childbirth, and avoidance of unintended pregnancies, and absence and avoidance of sexually transmitted infections, including HIV.

Hepatitis - A disease or condition (as hepatitis A or hepatitis B) marked by inflammation of the liver.

Hereditary - Genetically transmitted or transmittable from parent to offspring.

Heroin - A strongly physiologically addictive narcotic $C_{21}H_{23}NO_5$ that is made by acetylation of but is more potent than morphine and that is prohibited for medical use in the United States but is used illicitly for its euphoric effects.

Hidden illness - A hidden illness is a condition or disease whose symptoms aren't apparent to the outside world.

Hippocampus - An anatomical subdivision of the brain.

Hoarders – Those suffering with Schizophrenia, believing something bad will happen to them if they throw things away.

Homicidal tendencies - Having a tendency toward killing another human being.

Huntington's disease - a progressive neurodegenerative disorder that is inherited as an autosomal dominant trait, that usually begins in middle age, that is characterized especially by choreiform movements, emotional disturbances, and mental deterioration leading to dementia, and that is accompanied by atrophy of the caudate nucleus and the loss of certain brain cells with a decrease in the level of several neurotransmitters—called also Huntington's, Huntington's chorea.

Hydrocodone - A habit-forming compound derived from codeine and administered in the form of its bitartrate, usually in combination with other drugs such as an analgesic or cough sedative.

Hydromorphone - A ketone derived from morphine that is about five times as active biologically as morphine, and is administered in the form of its hydrochloride such as an analgesic.

Hypersexual behavior – Behavior that involves unusual or excessive concern with or indulgence in sexual activity.

Hypomania - A mood state characterized by persistent, and pervasive elevated (euphoric) or extreme happiness that is sometimes followed by an irritable mood, as well as thoughts and behaviors that are consistent with such a mood state.

Hypothyroidism - A state in which the thyroid gland does not produce a sufficient amount of the thyroid hormones thyroxine (T4) and triiodothyronine (T3).

Impulsive control disorder - A class of psychiatric disorders characterized by impulsivity – failure to resist a temptation, urge or impulse that may harm oneself or others. Many psychiatric disorders feature impulsivity, including substance-related disorders, attention deficit hyperactivity disorder, antisocial personality disorder, borderline personality disorder, conduct disorder, schizophrenia and mood disorders.

Impulsivity – A multifactorial construct that involves a tendency to act on a whim, displaying behavior characterized by little or no forethought, reflection, or consideration of the consequences

Infertility - Refers to the biological inability of a person to contribute to conception. Infertility may also refer to the state of a woman who is unable to carry a pregnancy to full term.

Information overload - Also known as infobesity or infoxication) refers to the difficulty a person can have understanding an issue and making decisions that can be caused by the presence of too much information.

Inherited traits - A distinguishing quality or characteristic that is transmitted genetically from one generation to the next.

Insomnia - Habitual sleeplessness; inability to sleep.

Instant messaging - A type of online chat that offers real-time text transmission over the Internet.

Internet addiction support - A social or support group that provide support to internet addicts.

Internet compulsions - Obsessive online gambling, shopping or day trading.

Interpersonal psychotherapy - A semi-structured treatment in which the patient. is educated about depression, and the Patient's relation to the environment, especially social functioning; unlike traditional psychotherapy, IP focuses on the present tense and not on underlying personality structures.

Interpersonal therapy - A kind of psychotherapy that views faulty communications, interactions, and interrelationships as basic factors in maladaptive behavior.

Interrelated factors - An element or cause that contributes to the making of a reciprocal relationship.

Intoxication - The state of being intoxicated, especially by alcohol.

Ipecac Syrup - An over-the-counter remedy made from the root of the Cephaelis ipecacuanha plant to induce vomiting.

Kleptomania - An obsessive impulse to steal regardless of economic need, usually arising from an unconscious symbolic value associated with the stolen item.

Lamotrigine - An anticonvulsant drug used in the treatment of epilepsy and bipolar disorder. It is also used off-label as an adjunct in treating clinical depression.[1] For epilepsy, it is used to treat focal seizures, primary and secondary tonic-clonic seizures, and seizures associated with Lennox-Gastaut syndrome. Like many other anticonvulsant medications, Lamotrigine also seems to act as an effective mood stabilizer, and has been the first U.S. Food and Drug Administration (FDA)-approved drug for this purpose since lithium, a drug approved almost 30 years earlier.

Line support group meeting – An on line meeting place that consist of condition-specific support groups, that offer patients regular social contact, accurate information and crucial emotional support.

Love addict anonymous – A fellowship of men and women whose common purpose is to recover from an unhealthy dependency on love, as it plays out in fantasies and relationships.

Low tar cigarettes - Cigarettes labeled as Lights, mild's, or Low-tar, and are considered to have a "lighter," less pronounced flavor than regular cigarettes. These cigarette brands may also contain lower levels of tar, nicotine, or other chemicals inhaled by the smoker. But are said to be no safer than regular cigarettes.

Low immune system - A state in which the immune system's ability to fight infectious disease is compromised or entirely absent. Immunodeficiency may also decrease cancer immunosurveillance.

LSD - A semisynthetic illicit organic compound derived from ergot that induces extreme sensory distortions, altered perceptions of reality, and intense emotional states, that may also produce delusions or paranoia, and that may sometimes cause panic reactions in response to the effects experienced.

Magnesium - A chemical element, with salts that are essential in nutrition, being required for the activity of many enzymes, especially those concerned with oxidative phosphorylation.

Major depression - A mental disorder characterized by a pervasive and persistent low mood that is accompanied by low self-esteem and by a loss of interest or pleasure in normally enjoyable activities.

Mania - An abnormally elated mental state, typically characterized by feelings of euphoria, lack of inhibitions, racing thoughts, diminished need for sleep, talkativeness, risk taking, and irritability. In extreme cases, mania can induce hallucinations and other psychotic symptoms.

Manic depression - Alternating moods of abnormal highs (mania) and lows (depression). Called bipolar disorder because of the swings between these opposing poles in mood. A type of depressive disease. Not nearly as prevalent as other forms of depressive disorders.

Mental disorders - Also called a mental illness or psychiatric disorder, is a mental or behavioral pattern or anomaly that causes either suffering or an impaired ability to function in ordinary life (disability), and which is not developmentally or socially normative. Mental disorders are generally defined by a combination of how a person feels, acts, thinks or perceives.

Mental health indicator – Tools used to obtain an assessment of the overall positive mental health (mental wellbeing) of the general population.

Mepridine - Used to relieve moderate to severe pain.

Message boards - An online discussion site where people can hold conversations in the form of posted messages. They differ from chat rooms in that messages are often longer than one line of text, and are at least temporarily archived.

Methadone - An addictive narcotic drug used especially in the form of its hydrochloride for the relief of pain and as a substitute narcotic in the treatment of heroin addiction.

Mixed episodes - A condition during which features of mania and depression, such as agitation, anxiety, fatigue, guilt, impulsiveness, irritability, morbid or suicidal ideation, panic, paranoia, pressured speech and rage, occur simultaneously.

Mood interrupters – Different types of disorders that make up bipolar disorder, which include mania, hypomania, depression, and mixed episodes, and each one has a very distinct set of symptoms.

Mood stabilizer - A psychiatric medication used to treat mood disorders characterized by intense and sustained mood shifts, typically bipolar disorder.

Multiple personality disorder – A mental disorder on the dissociative spectrum characterized by at least two distinct and relatively enduring identities or dissociated personality states that alternately control a person's behavior, and is accompanied by memory impairment for important information not explained by ordinary forgetfulness.

Naloxone - A potent antagonist of narcotic drugs and especially morphine that is administered in the form of its hydrochloride.

Naltrexone - An opioid receptor antagonist used primarily in the management of alcohol dependence and opioid dependence.

Neologisms - A newly coined term, word, or phrase, that may be in the process of entering common use, but has not yet been accepted into mainstream language.

Network support - A group of people who provide emotional and practical help to someone in serious difficulty.

Neurotransmitters - A substance in the body that carries a signal from one nerve cell to another.

Nicotine - A poisonous alkaloid that is the chief active principle of tobacco and that is used as an insecticide.

Nonparaphilic - Sexual addictions that are defined as repetitive sexual acts involving conventional, normative, or non-deviant sexual thoughts or behaviors that the person feels compelled or driven to perform, which may or may not cause distress. Nonparaphilic sexual addictions are not formally described in the DSM; however, a diagnosis of impulse-control disorder not otherwise specified (NOS) may be given if a person with this behavioral pattern experiences an interference in functioning (e.g. relationships, work, etc.) for at least six months.

Obsessive Compulsive Disorder - A psychoneurotic disorder in which the patient is beset with obsessions or compulsions or both and suffers extreme anxiety or depression through failure to think the obsessive thoughts or perform the compelling acts.

Obsessive masturbation - A condition in which a person feels compelled to masturbate in inappropriate situations. Compulsive masturbation is sometimes a sign of a sex addiction, mental health problem, or negative reaction to a prescription medication. A person with a sex addiction derives little to no pleasure from having sex, but compulsively participates in sexual acts anyway.

Obsessive thoughts - The hallmark of obsessive-compulsive disorder, but there are types of "obsessive" thoughts that are present in a variety of anxiety disorders that won't necessarily cause a diagnosis of OCD.

Opioids - Possessing some properties characteristic of opiate narcotics but not derived from opium.

Opioid withdrawal - An acute state caused by withdrawal of opioid narcotics from a person addicted to narcotics Clinical Sweating, shaking, headache, craving, vomiting, abdominal cramping, diarrhea, insomnia, confusion, agitation, other behavioral changes.

Osteoarthritis - Also known as degenerative arthritis or degenerative joint disease or osteoarthrosis, is a group of mechanical abnormalities involving degradation of joints,[1] including articular cartilage and subchondral bone.

Osteoporosis - A progressive bone disease that's characterized by a decrease in bone mass and density and that leads to an increased risk of fracture.

Overeaters anonymous - Offers a program of recovery from compulsive overeating, binge eating and other eating disorders using the Twelve Steps and Twelve Traditions of OA. Worldwide meetings and other tools provide a fellowship of experience, strength and hope where members respect one another's anonymity. OA charges no dues or fees; it is self-supporting through member contributions.

Oxycodone - An opioid analgesic derived from morphine

Oxycontin - A trademark for the drug oxycodone.

Panic disorder - An anxiety disorder characterized by recurrent unexpected panic attacks followed by a month or more of worry about their recurrence, implications, or consequences or by a change in behavior related to the panic attacks.

Paranoia - An unfounded or exaggerated distrust of others, sometimes reaching delusional proportions.

Paraphilias - A pattern of recurring sexually arousing mental imagery or behavior that involves unusual and especially socially unacceptable sexual practices (such as sadism, masochism, fetishism, or pedophilia).

Paraphilic - Any of a group of psychosexual disorders characterized by sexual fantasies, feelings, or activities involving a nonhuman object, a non-consenting partner such as a child, or pain or humiliation of oneself or one's partner. Also called sexual deviation.

Paroxetine - An antidepressant drug that acts by preventing the re-uptake after release of serotonin in the brain, thereby prolonging its action: used for treating depression, obsessive-compulsive disorders, and panic disorder.

Pedophilia - The act or fantasy on the part of an adult of engaging in sexual activity with a child or children.

Perimenopause - The period of a woman's life shortly before the occurrence of the menopause.

Personality trait - A stable and characteristic aspect of one's personality as a discrete manifestation of a set of values, beliefs, thoughts, attitudes, intentions, feelings, or actions.

Phobia - An extreme or irrational fear of or aversion to something.

Physical abandonment – While child abandonment typically involves physical abandonment - such as leaving a child at a stranger's doorstep when no one is home -- it may also include extreme cases of emotional abandonment -- such as when a "work-a-holic" parent offers little or no physical contact or emotional support over long periods of time

Physical abuse - An act of another party involving contact intended to cause feelings of physical pain, injury, or other physical suffering or bodily harm

Physical addiction - Drug dependence in which the drug is used to prevent withdrawal symptoms or in which it is associated with tolerance, or both.

Physical assault - An intentional act by one person that creates an apprehension in another of an imminent harmful or offensive contact.

Pornography - Sexually explicit erotic writings and images.

Post partum depression - A type of clinical depression that can affect women, and less frequently men, typically after childbirth.

Post traumatic stress disorder - A disorder that occurs among survivors of severe environmental stress such as a tornado, an airplane crash, or military combat. Symptoms include anxiety, insomnia, flashbacks, and nightmares. Patients with PTSD are unnecessarily vigilant; they may experience survivor guilt, and they sometimes cannot concentrate or experience joy.

Potassium - A mineral found in foods. It is also an electrolyte, which conducts electrical impulses throughout the body. It assists in a range of essential body functions, including: blood pressure.

Premenstrual dysphoric - A severe form of premenstrual syndrome, afflicting 3% to 8% of women.

Premenstrual syndrome - A collection of emotional symptoms, with or without physical symptoms, related to a woman's menstrual cycle.

Problem gambling - An urge to continuously gamble despite harmful negative consequences or a desire to stop. Problem gambling often is defined by whether harm is experienced by the gambler or others, rather than by the gambler's behavior.

Promiscuity - Miscellaneous mingling or selection of persons or things.

Purging - Consuming a large amount of food in a short amount of time, followed by an attempt to rid oneself of the food consumed typically by vomiting, taking a laxative, diuretic, or stimulant, and/or excessive exercise, because of an extensive concern for body weight.

Psychiatrist - A physician with additional medical training and experience in the diagnosis, prevention, and treatment of mental disorders.

Psychiatric nurse - The specialty field of a nurse that cares for people of all ages with mental illness or mental distress, such as schizophrenia, bipolar disorder, psychosis, depression or dementia. Nurses in this area receive more training in psychological therapies, building a therapeutic alliance, dealing with challenging behavior, and the administration of psychiatric medicine.

Psychodynamic therapy - A form of depth psychology, the primary focus of which is to reveal the unconscious content of a client's psyche in an effort to alleviate psychic tension.

Psychological - Knowledge that is often applied to the assessment and treatment of mental health problems, it is also directed towards understanding and solving problems in many different spheres of human activity.

Psychologist – One who evaluates, diagnoses, treats, and studies behavior and mental processes. Some psychologists, such as clinical and counseling psychologists, provide mental health care, and some psychologists, such as social or organizational psychologists conduct research and provide consultation services.

Psychotic – A person exhibiting the characteristics of a psychosis.

Re-attribute - Realize that the power and invasiveness of the thoughts you have are the result of OCD, which is most likely linked to a biochemical imbalance in your brain. Tell yourself, this isn't me it's my OCD, in an effort to remind yourself that the thoughts, and urges you have from OCD doesn't mean anything, and that they are just false messages coming from your brain.

Recovery groups - Voluntary associations of people who share a common desire to overcome drug addiction. Different groups use different methods, ranging from completely secular to explicitly spiritual. One survey of members found active involvement in any addiction recovery group correlates with higher chances of maintaining sobriety.

Recovery program - A course of treatment for people who are addicted to drugs or alcohol.

Re-focus – Work around the thoughts you have as a result of OCD, by directing your attention to another area or subject for at least a few moments. Do something different. Tell yourself that what you're experiencing is simply a symptom of OCD, and that you need to take part in other activities.

Re-label - Recognize that the obsessive thoughts, and desires that invade your mind are caused by OCD. An example is training yourself to say things like, I don't believe my hands are dirty, I don't really need to wash my hands, or what I'm sensing is only a compulsive urge to wash my hand.

Re-value - Don't take your thoughts that are associated with OCD at face value, because they are not important. Say things like, this is just that dumb obsession of mines, and it doesn't mean anything. It's all in my mind, and there is no reason for me to pay these thoughts any attention. Keep in mind, you may not be able to make the thought go away, but you don't have to entertain it either.

Ruptured esophagus - A rupture of the esophageal wall. 56% of esophageal perforations are iatrogenic, usually due to medical instrumentation such as an endoscopy or paraesophageal surgery.

Salivation - The act or process of secreting saliva.

Schizoid personality disorder - A personality disorder marked by indifference to social relationships and restricted range of emotional experience and expression.

Schizophrenia - A psychotic disorder (or a group of disorders) marked by severely impaired thinking, emotions, and behaviors.

Second-hand smoke - Smoke from burning tobacco products to which a person is unintentionally exposed, most commonly in the home, and formerly in public places.

Sedation - The act of calming by administration of a sedative.

Seizures - A single episode of epilepsy, often named for the type it represents.

Self-harm - The practice of cutting or otherwise wounding oneself, usually considered as indicating psychological disturbance.
Self-loathing - Hatred, disregard, and denigration of oneself.

Self-soothe - To bring tranquility or relief to oneself.

Serontoninergic (SSRI) - Any chemical that functions to enhance the effects mediated by serotonin in the body.

Sertraline - A drug that functions as an SSRI and is administered orally in the form of its hydrochloride $C_{17}H_{17}NCl_2 \cdot HCl$, especially to treat depression, anxiety, panic disorder, and obsessive-compulsive disorder.

Sex addiction – progressive intimacy disorder, characterized by compulsive sexual thoughts and acts

Sex addicts anonymous - A fellowship of recovering addicts, that offers a message of hope to anyone who suffers from sex addiction.

Sexaholics anonymous - A fellowship of men and women who share their experience, strength, and hope with each other that they may solve their common problem and help others to recover.

Sexual assault - Any involuntary sexual act in which a person is threatened, coerced, or forced to engage against their will, or any non-consensual sexual touching of a person. This includes rape (such as forced vaginal, anal or oral penetration or drug facilitated sexual assault), groping, forced kissing, child sexual abuse, or the torture of the victim in a sexual manner.

Sexual disorder - Any disorder involving sexual functioning, desire, or performance.

Sexual gratification – Sexual pleasure.

Skin picking - Also known as excoriation (skin-picking) disorder, neurotic excoriation, pathologic skin picking (PSP), compulsive skin picking (CSP) or psychogenic excoriation) is an impulse control disorder characterized by the repeated urge to pick at one's own skin, often to the extent that damage is caused.

Sleep apnea - A type of sleep disorder characterized by pauses in breathing or instances of shallow or infrequent breathing during sleep.

Sleep deprivation - The condition of not having enough sleep; it can be either chronic or acute.

Smoking cessation - Public health temporary or permanent halting of habitual cigarette smoking; withdrawal therapies; e.g., hypnosis, psychotherapy, group counseling, exposing smokers to patients with terminal lung cancer and nicotine chewing gum are often ineffective.

So-called negative symptoms – signifies that normal behaviors have disappeared, and are no longer evident in people that are healthy.

Social anxiety disorder - Also known as social phobia, is the most common anxiety disorder, and is also one of the most common psychiatric disorders, with 12% of American adults having experienced it in their lifetime.

Social factors - The facts and experiences that influence individuals' personality, attitudes and lifestyle.

Social network - A network of social interactions and personal relationships.

Social support - The perception and actuality that one is cared for, has assistance available from other people, and that one is part of a supportive social network.

Sodium - A soft, silver-white, chemically active metallic element that occurs naturally only in combination: a necessary element in the body for the maintenance of normal fluid balance and other physiological functions.

Split personalities - Is sometimes used to describe the psychiatric diagnosis Dissociative identity disorder. Sometimes people use it to refer to schizophrenia. Therefore, it is a non-technical term without a definition, and should not be used at all.

Sporadic - Occurring at irregular intervals; having no pattern or order in time.

Stimulant - A substance that temporarily increases the physiologic activity of an organ or organ system.

Stress - A state of mental tension and worry caused by problems in your life, work, etc.

Stress overload - Excessive amounts and types of demands that require action, is a human response that is experienced as a problem and contributes to the development of other problems.

Stress reduction techniques - Structured relaxation techniques to help control stress and improve your physical and mental well being.

Stress related disorder - A conscious or unconscious psychological feeling or physical situation which comes after as a result of physical or/and mental 'positive or negative pressure' to overwhelm adaptive capacities.

Substance abuse - Excessive use of a potentially addictive substance, especially one that may modify body functions, such as alcohol and drugs. Also called chemical abuse.

Substance related disorder - A patterned use of a substance (drug) in which the user consumes the substance in amounts or with methods that is harmful to themselves or others.

Sudden infant death syndrome - The unexplained death without warning of an apparently healthy infant, usually during sleep.

Tantrum - A fit of bad temper.

Temporal lobe - The lowest of the major subdivisions of the cortical mantle of the brain containing the sensory center for hearing, and forming the rear two thirds of the ventral surface of the cerebral hemisphere. It is separated from the frontal and parietal lobes above it by the fissure of Sylvius.

Therapy - The treatment of disease.

Thyroid issues - Inflammation of the thyroid, usually from a viral infection or autoimmune condition.

Tic disorder - Characterized by the persistent presence of tics, which are abrupt, repetitive involuntary movements and sounds that have been described as caricatures of normal physical acts. The best known of these disorders is Tourette's disorder, or Tourette's syndrome.

Tolerance - The capacity to absorb a drug continuously or in large doses without adverse effect; diminution in the response to a drug after prolonged use.

Topamax - An anticonvulsant (anti-epilepsy) drug that was recently approved for weight loss by the FDA in combination with phentermine.

Topiramate - An anticonvulsant (anti-epilepsy) drug, and was most recently approved for weight loss by the FDA in combination with phentermine.

Traumatic focused cognitive behavior therapy - A psychosocial treatment model designed to treat posttraumatic stress and related emotional and behavioral problems in children and adolescents.

Tremors – The shakes caused by withdrawal from drug dependency.

Trigger - Anything, as an act or event that initiates or precipitates a reaction or series of reactions.

Twelve-step program - Any program modeled after the 12-step self-help-group program used by Alcoholics Anonymous for rehabilitating alcoholics; central to all such programs is the belief in a God, transpersonal spiritual form of energy or superhuman power.

Vicodin - A controlled substance, which is a ketone derivative of codeine that is about six times more potent than codeine.

Vitamin deficiencies - A state or condition resulting from the lack of or inability to use one or more vitamins

Voyeurism - A person who derives sexual gratification from observing the naked bodies or sexual acts of others, especially from a secret vantage point.

Washers – those fearful of being polluted, and have an urge to clean things or wash their hands.

Withdrawal - Those side effects experienced by a person who has become physically dependent on a substance, upon decreasing the substance's dosage or discontinuing its use.

Worry period – Time set aside once or twice every day, lasting 10 each time, that one can dedicate to obsessing.

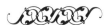

ABOUT THE AUTHOR

Evangelist Dolores Roberson Jackson was born to John and Leana Roberson on September 11, 1961 in Detroit Michigan. She is the seventh of their 10 children, and currently resides in Clinton Township, Michigan. Evangelist Jackson is the mother of one child Keana Roberson, and enjoys being a grandmother to four grandchildren, Iyana Simone, Imani Danielle, Immanuel Yeshua, and Ilana Gabrielle. She is a Spirit-filled, born again believer who gave her life to the Lord in 1994. She has a great love for people, and enjoys helping people in any way she can. She is also passionate about preaching and teaching the word of God.

Her special love for ministry work began when she started teaching bible study classes at General Motors, Warren Power Train plant in 1998. There, Evangelist Jackson ministered, and witnessed to many co-workers, and along with other preachers, helped run a two-week revival which was held during both shifts, something that is unheard of in other workplaces. And it was during that year that she received her call to ministry.

She attended and graduated with the very first class from the School of Ministry at Perfecting church in Detroit, Michigan, while under the leadership of Pastor Marvin L. Winans. She became a licensed and ordained Evangelist while under the leadership of Apostle Donald Coleman at New Breakthrough Church in Detroit, Michigan., in 2007. She attended Ashland Theological Seminary and graduated in 2010 with a degree of Practical Ministry. She currently attends King of Kings International Church where she serves under Bishop Willie M Thornton. She heads up the Prison Ministry, is part of the Evangelism Ministry and is also a Worship Leader with the Praise Team.

Evangelist Jackson writes with much love for God's people, aiming to bring about an awareness of where the church is and where God desires to take it. Through her books, she hopes to provide insight on what we, the body of Christ can do to prepare for the second coming of Christ Jesus, and also help people successfully navigate through their lives. Dolores is employed with General Motors Corporation, where she has been a dedicated employee for over 30 years and is also an entrepreneur. She loves to sing, and has written many beautiful gospel songs. She also writes poetry, creates unique greeting cards, and is the founder of WIC Resource and Development Center, My Brother's Keeper Supportive Housing and Leading Today's Youth; A mentoring and etiquette program for youth ages 7 to 18.

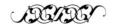